EFFICACY OF WARM FOOT BATH AMONG CHILDREN

SMT. BEDRE SUWARNA SHRIRAM

CONTENTS

CHAPTER I

PROLOGUE

A good night's sleep is one in which you fall asleep quickly, do not fully wake up during the night, do not wake up too early, and wake up feeling refreshed. It is not usual for healthy adults of any age to have trouble falling asleep or sleeping through the night on a regular basis. However, not everyone needs the same amount of sleep, and the quality of sleep varies with age.

Adults and teenagers sleep more soundly than young children and the elderly. Over a person's lifespan, the amount of time spent in deep sleep stages varies. Infants and toddlers require far more sleep than older children and adults. Most children have adult-like sleep patterns by the time they reach the age of five: they are awake during the day and then sleep through the night. Until the age of 80, the quantity of time spent sleeping gradually declines.

Sleep cycles usually repeat every 90 to 110 minutes. Each cycle is made up of a sequence of different sleep phases. There are two main types of sleep: REM sleep, NON -REM sleep. The acronym REM stands for "rapid eye movement." This moniker refers to the rapid eye movements that occur during deep slumber. When toddlers and adults sleep deeply, their eyes move rapidly back and forth while their eyelids stay closed. Only during the REM stages can we dream.

There are several ideas regarding what constitutes regular sleep and how it varies with age. Sleep onset, or the time required to enter light sleep, is known to increase with age. However, the age-related variation is minor: the length of sleep onset rises by less than ten minutes on average between the ages of 20 and 80.

Between the ages of five and nineteen, the stages of profound REM sleep increase longer. They then remain rather steady until they reach the age of 60. Ones over the age of 60 have somewhat less deep sleep and do not sleep as well as younger people.

A night's sleep of nine hours is considered typical for youngsters aged five to twelve. Around the age of 40, the average individual sleeps about seven hours per night, and between the ages of 55 and 60, they sleep about six and a half hours each night. A healthy 80-year-old sleeps around six hours every night on average. However, these are just averages; each person requires a different amount of sleep. Sleep has an impact on how children feel and operate. Assisting the kid in getting the required amount of sleep by enhancing the child's health, psychological well-being, and safety. Sleep is essential for a child's growth and development, as well as his or her capacity to study. Individual variances may exist between children, with preschool-aged children needing 1012 hours and school-aged children requiring at least 9 hours. Teenagers require more sleep than adults. Adequate sleep is an essential component of living a healthy lifestyle. During sleep, the body and brain actively collaborate to maintain optimal brain and body function. Sleep aids a child's ability to focus and recall what he or she has learned. Sleep helps to boost memory.

Sleeping appears to help with learning, almost as if it were more practises. Sleeping properly, for example, strengthens the immune system, which aids in the battle against infections, and so may reduce your child's chance of becoming ill. Even missing an hour of sleep every night on a regular basis might have a negative impact on a child's performance. This is due to the fact that such regular sleep deprivation mounts up and creates a sleep debt. With each additional night of sleep loss, performance and function deteriorate.[1]

Being in the hospital is associated with sleep disruptions for many children with medical difficulties. For example, 25% of cancer-affected children in hospitals reported sleep issues such fragmentation and nocturnal awakening. Sleep problems can be caused by disruptions in routine, anxiety and concerns about separation from parents, a lack of privacy, and frequent interruptions by medical staff. Children may need to adjust their sleeping position as a result of IV insertion or surgical incision placement.

Melatonin is a hormone produced by the pineal gland that has a daily rhythm that is influenced by light: light inhibits melatonin release, whilst darkness enhances it. Melatonin has a chronobiological as well as a sleep-inducing function. Exogenous melatonin therapy improves sleep efficiency and overall sleep duration while decreasing sleep latency. Melatonin also aids in the restoration of a messed-up circadian rhythm. Melatonin aids in the preservation of healthy sleep architecture by promoting sleep in a manner similar to that of the natural sleep process. Melatonin has been demonstrated to aid children with sleep issues, and it is routinely used in paediatric sleep clinics across the world to treat insomnia and other sleep disorders. Melatonin has a minimal number of adverse effects. Circadian is a slow-release melatonin formulation that mimics natural melatonin secretion at night. Sleep latency and total sleep time improved in children with sleep disorders who were treated with controlled release melatonin.

In our daily lives, sleep is just as important as water and food. Even though we believe sleep just relaxes our exhausted body, our brain stays working all night. Sleep is necessary for mental and physical health.

Your body undergoes a number of changes when you sleep, allowing you to get the rest you need. These changes help your body to repair and restore itself. Because the brain and the body are able to recover and heal when we sleep, we experience enhanced physical and mental performance the following day as well as throughout time. When you don't get enough sleep, these vital functions are disrupted, impacting your mood, thinking, energy levels, and concentration. As a consequence, obtaining enough sleep is critical adults need 7 to 9 hours of sleep, while children and teenagers need even more.

During an ordinary night's sleep, your body will go through four or five cycles of sleep. Every sleep cycle has four phases. The REM (rapid eye movement) phase of sleep and the non-REM phase of sleep have subdivided further into two categories within the four stages of sleep. These contrasts are essential due to the fact that the processes that take place during REM sleep are considerably diverse from those that take place within non-REM sleep. Non-REM sleep activity dominates the first three phases of sleep. Stage 1 is a brief period that corresponds to becoming sleepy and drifting off. As you go asleep, your body and mind begin to slow down. The first two phases are the easiest to break free from. The body is in recuperation mode and slows down even further within Stage 3, sometimes called as deep sleep. Simultaneously, overall brain activity declines, and activity pulses occur, which helps prevent undesired awakenings. REM sleep is the fourth stage of sleep.

The most vivid dreams are associated with REM phases because they enable brain activity to spike. At levels comparable to being awake. During REM sleep, our heart rate and breathing rate increase, but most of our muscles stay still, preventing us from carrying out our imaginations. A sleep cycle might last anywhere from 70 to 120 minutes. The beginning sleep cycles of the nights are characterized by a larger proportion of non-REM sleep than REM sleep. The REM sleep stage typically begins sometime in the middle of the night's second half. Sleep architecture refers to the order in which sleep stages and cycles occur during a specific sleep period. [2]

Circadian rhythms and sleep drive are the two fundamental systems that control sleep. A biological clock housed in the brain regulates circadian rhythms. One of the key roles of the clock is to respond to light signals by raising melatonin production at night and shutting it off when it senses light. Because they are unable to notice and react to these light signals, those who are completely blind have difficulty sleeping. The urge to sleep, like the want to eat, is vital. During the day, your need to sleep becomes stronger, and you must sleep when it reaches a particular level.

A fundamental contrast among sleep and hunger is as follows: Whether you're at a meeting or driving, your body could make you eat once you're hungry, or it might also make you sleep when you're tired. When you're tired, your body may enter micro sleep while your eyes are open. Napping for more than 30 minutes in the afternoon may reduce your sleep drive.3

Almost every part of the body experiences major modifications when sleeping. As you sleep, your brain's neurons transform from active to passive, sending messages across your body. Sleep boosts the cardiovascular and immunological systems and regulates metabolism, according to study. During sleep, significant changes in critical biological activities may be identified.

Breathing: Non-REM sleep lowers breathing, while deep sleep stage 3 has the lowest respiratory rates. REM sleep causes erratic breathing.

Heart Rate: Stage 1 heart rate decreases and reaches a low in Stage 3. REM sleep quickens the pulse to nearly awake levels.

Muscle Tone: As non-REM sleep develops, muscles relax and energy consumption drops. During REM, atonia paralyses most muscles. This prevents flailing legs and arms from dream material. Respiratory and ocular muscles remain active, with quick eye movement. Sleep's name comes from eyes darting under closed eyelids. [4]

Brain Activity: Brain waves indicate various patterns for each sleep stage when recorded. In early non-REM sleep, brain waves drop substantially, but in Stages 2 and 3 there remain short bursts of activity. REM sleep enhances brain activity, causing distinct brain waves. Vivid dreams are caused by enhanced brain activity during REM sleep. Non-REM sleep is supposed to support optimal brain function while awake, even with diminished brain activity.

Dreaming: REM sleep is when dreaming is most common and powerful REM dreams are more innovative, immersive, and unusual than non-REM dreams.[5]

Hormone Levels: Sleep and circadian rhythm regulate hormone synthesis, including:

- Melatonin, a sleep-inducing hormone.
- Growth hormone helps bone, muscle development and metabolism.
- Cortisol a body stress hormone
- The appetite-controlling hormones leptin and ghrelin

Different phases of sleep affect hormone levels, and Sleep quality affects daily hormone synthesis. [6]

Paediatric patients typically have sleep disturbance, which affects both the kid and the parent. Paediatric patients in critical care units, for example, may lose up to 54 percent of their sleep hours.[7] whereas children in regular paediatric units can lose 20 percent to 25 percent of their sleep hours [8].

According to science, taking a warm footbath before bed may help you shift from awake to sleep faster by lowering core temperature and increasing distal (hands and feet) temperature. It may also help you sleep better; allowing you to wake up feeling refreshed and rejuvenated the following day. [9]

The current study is important as sleep problem in hospitalized children is big issue. To find out non pharmacologic solution like footbath is efficacious or not hence the aim of this research is to assess efficacy of warm foot bath in promotion of early sleep onset among hospitalized children.

CHAPTER II

REVIEW OF LITERATURE

Review of literature is an overview of the previously works on specific topic. The term can refer to a full scholarly paper or a section of a scholarly work such as a book, or an article. An attempt has been made in this study to review related literature on the selected topic

Search Strategy

Definition: A search strategy is defined as an organized structure of the key terms that are being used to search a database. The search strategy combines the key concepts of the search question of a researcher in order to retrieve accurate results for the study.

A well-constructed search strategy can be defined as the core of the systematic review that can report in the methods section of the paper. The search strategy can retrieve a majority of the studies that can help the researcher to assess for the studies that fulfils the eligibility & inclusion for the study. The quality of the search strategy is also observed to affect the items that may have been missed.

In this research, the researcher follows the stepwise search strategy to gain more knowledge and more articles and literatures for supporting the present research study "Efficacy of warm foot bath in early onset of sleep among hospitalized children using PRISMA format. The research searched for the supportive researches by using search engines like PUBMED, MEDLINE, MESH, RESEARCH GATE, CINAHL, etc.

CONCISE SYSTEMATIC REVIEW OF LITERATURE

(PRISMA FLOW DIAGRAM)

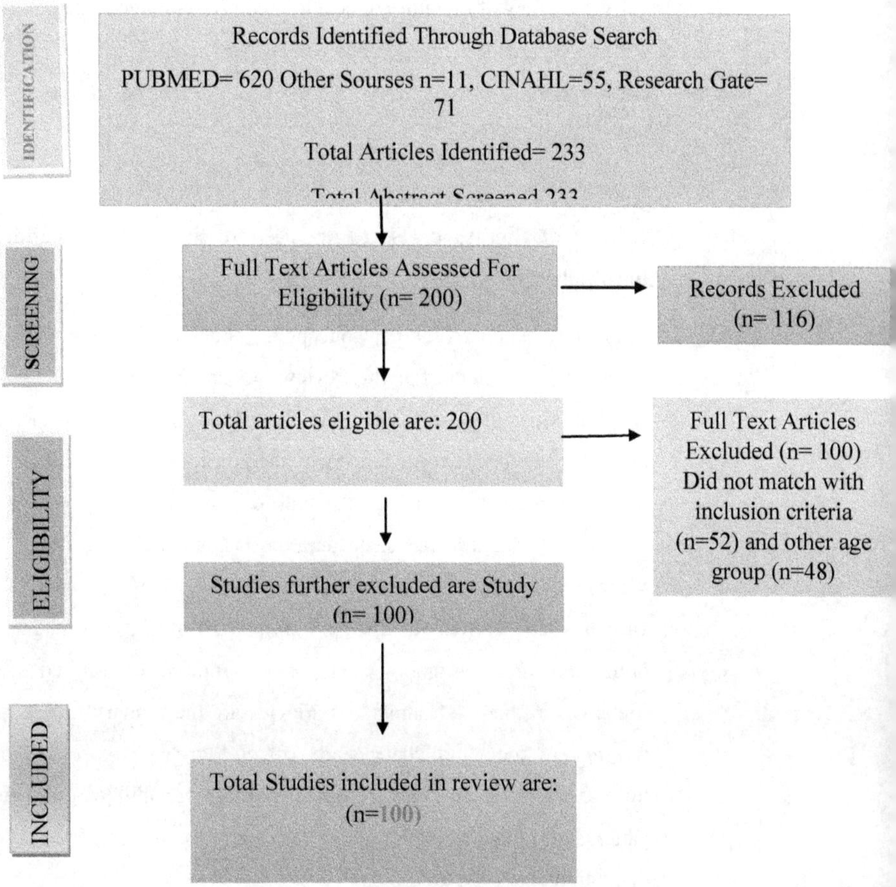

Figure1: Prisma Flow Diagram

The researcher did an extensive search of existing literature, and organized it under following heading:

- Review of literature related to sleep disturbances of children at hospitalization.
- Review of literature related to Sleep Assessment scale
- Review of literature related to BEARS scale
- Review of literature related to effectiveness of Warm foot bath on early onset of sleep

Review of literature related to sleep disturbances of children during hospitalization

This study conducted as per conceptual model of sleep problems in children admitted to hospitals. For this review, 45 papers were included. Despite the fact that most sleep difficulties are caused by environmental factors (such as noise and staff interruptions), most therapies focused on the child utilising relaxation methods. Although the bulk of the therapies were tiny pilot trials, early results suggest that sleep duration is improved. The Pediatric Inpatient Sleep Model was developed to show how sleep disorders, sleep-related variables, and current therapeutic components are linked. Larger-scale sleep promotion therapies among hospitalised children are required in replication trials. Given that environmental variables are the primary source of nocturnal waking, environmental changes are critical. More study is needed to determine the factors that contribute to intra individual variability in interrupted sleep patterns during hospitalizations, as well as the repercussions of this disruptions.[10]

A study reported scoping review of sleep in hospitalised children and adolescents. Short sleep is a danger for hospitalised children and adolescents, with negative health consequences, but little is known about real sleep length, the variables that induce sleep disruptions in a paediatric inpatient environment, and what has been done to encourage sleep in this group. Looked through five electronic databases (PubMed, CENTRAL, CINAHL, PsycINFO, and Scopus), and just 28 of the 3770 references found were relevant. Study discovered that four out of nineteen studies reporting age-specific sleep durations came within the National Sleep Foundation's guidelines for age-specific sleep durations. External influences, such as nursing care activities and noise from equipment and other patients, were the most often reported reasons of sleep disruptions. Patients, parents, and healthcare professionals tended to approve of sleep-promoting therapies. The research in this field, however, is inconsistent in terms of technique, reporting, and demographic characteristics. The results underscore the necessity of prioritising and enhancing sleep in paediatric patients in hospitals, as well as the need for uniformity in the planning and reporting of research in this sector.[11]

A Study conducted on the effects of hospitalisation on children's sleep patterns, regardless of previous sleep issues. Patients with PSP had an average increase of one hour in total sleep hours per day, which improved their sleep pattern. The total hours of sleep decreased in patients without PSP, but the time it took to fall asleep, the frequency of daytime naps, and nocturnal awakenings all rose. Sleep disruptions were linked to the sound of alarms, the presence of venous catheters and tubes, and the arrival and leave of healthcare staff into the rooms. Hospitalization disrupts sleep habits, particularly in children who have never had sleep issues before. They urge that all hospitalised children's sleep habits be investigated and that external variables linked with their disruption be minimised as much as feasible.[12]

A Study to develop an evidence-based guideline for nurses to promote sleep for hospitalised children. There were 61 adult-centric suggestions included in the existing relevant guidelines. Following changes to the evidence base, six composited recommendations were developed to help children sleep in hospitals: prioritising patient safety; collaborating with the mother or caregiver to promote sleep; coordinating the ward routine and environment to improve sleep; working with clinical and non-clinical staff; and performing basic sleep assessments. The nursing regulatory framework in South Africa was used to guide practise recommendations. For children, hospitalisation is a period of physiological and psychological deregulation, which is exacerbated by poor sleep. By applying this African-centric strategy in collaboration with moms, nurses may increase sleep during hospitalisation. [13]

Another study reported regarding sleep Disturbances in Paediatric Cancer Patients: Prevalence, Diagnosis, and Treatment Sleep disruptions are an understudied but widespread cause of concern among juvenile cancer patients and survivors, with negative consequences for their quality of life. Sleep problems are caused by a variety of circumstances, but identifying specific contributions is challenging, making it difficult to identify therapeutic targets. Disrupted sleep and its poor effect on quality of life persist in many juvenile cancer patients throughout adulthood, affecting numerous functional areas. The forms and incidence of sleep disruptions in paediatric cancer patients during active treatment and survivorship are highlighted in this study. The impact of cancer and its treatment, psychological and familial variables, as well as individual-patient characteristics such as genetics, mood, and coping abilities, are highlighted as potential etiological and risk factors for disturbed sleep. While the literature is evaluated for current evaluation and therapy options, considerable gaps in our knowledge of sleep disorders in paediatric cancer patients and survivors appear. The analysis finishes with suggestions for areas that need further investigation [14]

The study showed effect of parental mental health, child diet, and exercise in sleep disturbances in a sample of Lebanese children. A total of 76 youngsters (19%) reported sleep problems (PSQ scores of 8 or more). Greater paternal sadness (Beta = 0.079, p = 0.010), mother depression (Beta = 0.089, p = 0.001), and higher anxiety in the father (Beta = 0.064, p = 0.021) were significantly linked with higher PSQ scores (poor sleep) in the kid, according to the multivariable analysis. Lower PSQ scores were significantly linked with higher Family Nutrition and Physical Activity Screening Tool scores in the kid (Beta = -0.161, p 0.001). (better sleep). Children's sleeping difficulties were linked to paternal worry and depression, as well as mother sadness. Future research is required to determine the impact of parents on children's development.[15]

A cross-sectional research was done with 124 eligible youngsters who were approached for participation, 69 of whom agreed (35 [51 percent] female; 20 [29 percent] aged 1-3 years, 10 [14 percent] aged 4-7 years, 17 [24 percent] aged 8-12 years, and 22 [32 percent] aged 13-18 years; 58 [84 percent] in the general paediatric unit). Children aged 1 to 3, 4 to 7, 8 to 12, and 13 to 18 years old slept for an average of 444 (132), 475 (86), 436 (114), and 384 (83) minutes at night, with an average (SD) of 14 (3), 18 (3), 14 (8), and 12 (6) night awakenings, respectively. Chlldren in general pediatric units slept 258 minutes more per night than children in pediatric intensive care units (95 percent CI, 165.16-350.56 minutes; P.001), while children in for planned surgery slept 123 minutes more than children admitted for exacerbations of chronic illness. Clinicians, administrators, and hospital design specialists should collaborate to find solutions to the most common causes of overnight waking in hospitals.[16]

A Narrative Review of the Genetics of Sleep Disorders in Children Sleep is a ubiquitous, well-preserved mechanism that is necessary for human and animal survival but whose full roles are yet unknown. For various sleep disorders, familial recurrence is recognised, although definitive evidence is absent for many of them Furthermore, new knowledge on epigenetic gene-environment interactions is complicating our understanding of the genetic control of sleep and associated problems.[17]

The study was conducted regarding Lack of sleep in hospitalised children: causes and consequences. Sleep is an important function that accounts for a third of our lives. In the short and long term, sleep deprivation may cause medical and psychological problems. Hospitalization, regardless of the reason for admission, does not promote adequate and restorative sleep. Both environmental (light, noise) and internal (procedures, medications, and care) variables influence it. The critical care unit is where it is more difficult to fall asleep and stay asleep. This is in addition to the severity of the illness and its structural and functional properties. A lack of sleep, either in amount or quality, may lead to delirium, a condition of severe disorientation that often affects hospitalised children. The needed job is to promote a collaborative effort across all sectors of the hospital environment aimed at preserving sleep as much as feasible.[18]

Sleep characteristics are linked to obesity indicators. A total of 151 people were examined. Independent of age and gender, overweight/obese children exhibited substantially higher odds for arousal index (prepubertal children:

1.28, CI: 1.06, 1.67; pubertal children: 1.65, CI: 1.19, 2.29) than normal-weight children. After controlling for age and gender, arousal-index was shown to be favourably linked with C-peptide (r=0.30, p=0.01) and negatively associated with triglycerides (r=-0.34, p=0.005) in pre pubertal children. However, when accounting for body mass index standard deviation scores, the relationships were reduced (BMI-SDS). Independent of age, sex, or BMI-SDS, greater levels of apnoea -hypopnoea-index and pCO2 predicted increased lipoprotein (a) levels in pubertal children (r=0.35, p=0.03 and r=0.40, p=0.01, respectively). Study was concluded that overweight and obesity in children might affect sleep quality as judged by the arousal index, which should be taken into account in future intervention programmes. [19]

The study shows the length and disturbances of paediatric inpatient sleep. Patients slept 7 and 4 hours less in the hospital than at home among 246 patients (Newborn: 787 318 min at home vs. 354 211 min in hospital, p 0.001; Infants: 703 203 min at home vs. 412 152 min in hospital, p 0.01). When compared to NSF guidelines, newborn infants likewise had >2 h sleep deficits at home (Newborns: 787 318 min at home vs. 930 min recommended, p 0.05 The correlation between night-time traffic and caregiver-reported nightly awakenings was substantial (Spearman Rank Correlation Coefficient: 0.83, p 0.001). Both in the hospital and at home, hospitalisation is a squandered chance to enhance sleep. [20]

The study was conducted on Sleep and mood in paediatric medulloblastoma patients undergoing high-dose chemotherapy and hematopoietic rescue. With considerable between-subjects variability, sleep duration was short, sleep efficiency was low, and daytime napping was prevalent. During hospitalisation, patients with medulloblastoma are susceptible to sleep disturbances, and mood may be a significant factor to consider. Sleep and mood are two variables that may be addressed to improve daytime performance. [21]

One of the study reported comprehensive evaluation of sleep in paediatric cancer patients in hospitals. The participants (n = 147) varied in age from 1 to 18. When compared to previously establish age-related standards, data from objective and subjective sleep evaluations revealed that child sleep was interrupted in the hospital. Noise, light levels, and interruptions from the staff room were all linked to less overall sleep minutes and more nightly awakenings. The present study's methodological shortcomings, as well as future research directions, are explored. Investigations into the causes of increased sleep problems may be utilised to improve hospital operations in order to establish a more supportive sleep environment and more effective screening tools for patients who are at a higher risk of sleep problems. This might assist to reduce the role of hospitalisation in causing and sustaining persistent sleep problems in children with cancer. [22]

This study reported that Children's and parents' experiences in hospitals were investigated. Parents reported poor sleep quality for themselves and, to a lesser degree, their children. Noise and light, as well as ward routines, have been found as major sleep disruptors. Parents indicated that lack of sleep affected their own and their child's emotional control, impairing daytime parent-child connections. Furthermore, they said that sleep loss had a detrimental influence on their decision-making about their child's medical treatment.[23]

The researchers looked at the impact of hospitalisation on the sleep habits of newborns, infants, and toddlers, as well as mothers' perceptions of changes in their children's sleep patterns. Children under the age of two who had been in the hospital for more than two days were chosen at random for the study. To collect data, mothers were given an anonymous questionnaire containing open and closed questions. Two hundred and one children were participated in the study, with an average age of 11.2 months (SD 10.3). In the hospital, the number of children sleeping fewer than 5 hours per night climbed by 4.7 percent, while the number of children sleeping 9 to 11 hours per night declined by 5.9%. Mothers put their children to bed later in hospitals than at home. At the hospital, the number of people going to bed between 9 and 10 p.m. fell by 9.8%, while the number of youngsters going to bed between 10 and 11 p.m. rose by 10.1 percent. The number of children who had two to four nocturnal awakenings increased by 13.9 percent, while the number of children who experienced four to six nocturnal awakenings grew by 4.8 percent; 50.5 percent of mothers said that nurses disturbed their children's sleep to offer care. Even if their children were more disturbed and restless, mothers thought their children were getting enough sleep. Getting their children to sleep was more difficult for women with only one kid (P=0.02).[24]

A systematic review Research reported on Sleep Disturbances in Children with Chronic Fatigue Syndrome. Six studies were considered, the majority of which were case-controlled designs. Although the results varied across research, most revealed that children and adolescents with CFS had much greater sleep disruptions than healthy controls. There were significant methodological differences and limitations. The findings should be regarded with caution. "More research is needed to better understand the nature and extent of sleep disturbance in children with CFS, with a focus on (1) identifying the specific types, causes, and severity of sleep disturbances; (2) the specific consequences of sleep disturbances; and (3) the most effective sleep interventions in this population". [25]

The study evaluated the incidence of self-reported sleep disruption in children with a range of medical conditions admitted to a tertiary children's hospital. For one hospital inpatient night, 107 youngsters were polled. Overall, 52.3 percent of people had trouble sleeping. Further extensive research of particular causes of this condition was restricted due to the vast age range and diversity of diagnoses. This suggests that these children already had a problem sleeping before they were admitted to the hospital, since bad sleep before admission was the best predictor of poor sleep while in the hospital. Toileting (17.8%) or spontaneous awakenings were the most common causes of unprompted awakenings (17.8 percent). Nursing care (25.2 percent), alarms (12.1 percent), and discomfort were among the hospital-specific factors that awoke youngsters (12.1 percent). Children who are sick in the hospital have a higher prevalence of sleep problems compared to children who are well and living in the community.[26]

The study conducted on the Children's Report of Sleep Patterns (CRSP) is a school-aged child's self-reported sleep assessment. The CRSP was shown to be both reliable and valid. "Children who visited a sleep clinic or laboratory (vs. the general public), younger children (vs. older children), and children who slept less than 8 hours or whose sleep onset was later than 22:00 on actigraphy all exhibited varied sleep hygiene and sleep disruptions". "There was also a relationship between the CRSP and children's worry and exhaustion. Over 40% of parents were completely unaware that their children were experiencing sleep start delays, nocturnal waking, or poor sleep quality. The three modules of the CRSP may be used together or independently to examine sleep patterns, sleep hygiene, and sleep disturbances in children aged 8 to 12. Children not only give reliable information on their sleep, but they may also supply information that would be overlooked if just parental reports were utilised in clinical and research settings".[27]

The study conducted as night-time sleep disruptions, the hospital care environment, and symptoms in elementary school-age children with cancer. Sleep varied based on time of night ($F = 56.27$, $p < 0.01$), with sleep onset delayed past 10 pm. A basic mixed linear model identified significant fixed effects for sound ($F = 50.87$, $p < 0.01$) and light ($F = 7.04$, $p < 0.01$) on minutes of sleep. A backward regression model including sound, light, medication doses, pain, and nausea accounted for about 57% of the variance in sleep minutes ($F = 62.85$, $p < 0.01$). Sleep was marked by frequent awakenings, limiting children's ability to experience full sleep cycles. Multiple factors—in particular, excessive sound levels—compromise sleep quantity and quality throughout the night. [28]

A community-based study of "sleep and behaviour issues in children aged 12 to 36 months. Sleep issues reported by mothers were linked to children's behavioural problems at home, while nap problems reported by daycare workers were linked to children's behavioural problems at day-care. Behavioral difficulties reported by childcare workers were linked to behavioural problems reported by mothers. Mothers reported higher behavioural difficulties in older children in the sleep difficulty group. Children with sleep issues were less satisfied at day- care, according to day- care providers. Children who were happy after naps had fewer problems calming down at night. Children who had trouble falling asleep at day-care had greater behavioural issues, according to their mothers. Napping is an integral part of toddlers' sleep in childcare environments. The presence of crossover effects between children's sleep and behaviour at day-care and at home suggests that moms' and childcare providers' perspectives are comparable. The findings imply that talks concerning sleep issues and settling at home and in daycares occur between parents and daycare providers. Parents and childcare providers would benefit from learning more about the link between sleep and behavioural issues".[29]

The study showed Prevalence, "patterns and persistence of sleep problems in the first 3 years of life. Prevalence of a parent-reported sleep problem was 10% at all assessment intervals. Night waking and shorter sleep duration were associated with a parent-reported sleep problem during infancy and early toddlerhood (6–24 months), whereas nightmares and restless sleep emerged as associations with report of a sleep problem in later developmental periods (24–36 months). Prolonged sleep latency was associated with parent report of a sleep problem throughout the study period. In contrast, napping, sleep location, and snoring were not associated with parent-reported sleep problems. Twenty-one percent of children with sleep problems in infancy (compared with 6% of those without) had sleep problems in the third year of life. Ten percent of children are reported to have a sleep problem at any given point during early childhood, and these problems persist in a significant minority of children throughout early development. Parent response to a single-item nonspecific sleep query may overlook relevant sleep behaviours and symptoms associated with clinical morbidity".[30]

A study was conducted on children suffering with attention deficit hyperactivity disorder have sleep problems. Researchers argue in this article that in-depth questioning about sleepiness, sleep-disordered breathing, or problematic behaviours at bedtime, during the night, and upon awakening, As well as night-to-night sleep duration variability, is required for a better understanding and treatment of children who exhibit inattentive, hyperactive, impulsive behaviours. The connections between sleep and attention deficit hyperactivity disorder (ADHD) are complex, and they are frequently overlooked by practitioners. Restless sleep should be evaluated for restless legs syndrome or periodic limb movement disorder, and awakenings should be explored for parasomnias, dyssomnias, or sleep disorders, according to the findings of the study.[31]

In this study the importance of a model in understanding sleep-wake behaviour and sleep problems in children. The findings show that circadian and sleep homeostatic systems alter throughout time in the first two decades of life. Infancy's sleep-wake and crying behaviour may be influenced by the developmental interplay of both systems. Evidence suggests that the dynamics of sleep homeostatic mechanisms slow down throughout childhood (i.e., sleep pressure builds more slowly with age), allowing youngsters to stay awake for longer periods of time. Another hot issue right now is teenage sleep phase delay, which seems to be predominantly caused by maturational alterations in sleep homeostatic and circadian mechanisms. The two-process model of sleep regulation is a useful tool for analysing and forecasting sleep-wake behaviour in children. Such understanding is critical for better anticipatory advice, parental education, patient treatment, and the development of suitable social policies.[32]

A study was conducted related to sleep difficulties in newborns and young children. Approximately 25% of children under the age of 5 have a sleep issue. A considerable disturbance in the kid's sleep may occur, regardless of whether the issue is acute or chronic, and can have a detrimental influence on the child and family. This is the second part in a two-part series on baby and early child sleep. Sleep difficulties are examined in terms of its description, effect, and clinical assessment.[33]

The study despite that school-aged children's sleep and behavior issues the fact that 10.8% of the sample reported sleep issues in the previous six months, fewer than half of the parents who recognized sleep problems said they had addressed sleep with their child's physician. A history of sleep disorders before the age of two years was the strongest predictor of present sleep issues. Snoring, fatigue throughout the day, and requiring an inordinate amount of time to fall asleep were all highly prevalent, affecting over 20% of the overall sample on at least one night each week. The sleep difficulties questionnaire's component analysis revealed five sleep issue variables that accounted for 58.7% of the variation. The only sleep difficulty connected with age was enuresis/gags. This component was graded higher by younger youngsters. The length of naps was strongly linked to age and bedtimes throughout the week and on weekends. Younger children, as predicted, slept for longer lengths of time and went to bed sooner. In addition, naps and later bedtimes throughout the week and weekend were linked to greater weariness factor scores. Enuresis/gags scores were significantly greater in boys than in girls, and higher enuresis/gags scores were linked to a higher occurrence of trauma and falls. There was no link between bedtime and any other sleep difficulty component score. Children who scored high on weariness were more likely to have been hospitalized before.

The sleep habit of sharing a bed was highly connected with fatigue factor scores, but not with sharing a room. No sleep difficulty factor score was connected with sharing a room. Allergies, frequent falls, and sharing a bed were all linked to high noise sleep ratings. Children with high sleeplessness scores were also more likely to have a higher incidence of allergies. In school-aged children getting standard medical treatment, parental perceptions of global sleep disorders were unexpectedly prevalent. Parents' complaints of their children's sleep issues might be a warning indicator for particular sleep issues as well as psychological, social, or medical issues. Sleep difficulties should be discussed with school-aged children at pediatric checkups[34]

According to a study on sleep disorders and issues in children, Sleep disturbances are prevalent in children. There is a difference made between difficulties with abnormal polysomnography (such as parasomnias, sleep apnoea, and narcolepsy) and behavioural disorders with normal polysomnography. The parasomnias, which include sleep terrors, somnambulism, and enuresis, appear to be linked to CNS immaturity and are frequently outgrown. Physicians can be of considerable help to these families by advising to parents procedures that have been proven to work.[35]

Sleep patterns and sleep disruption in elementary school-aged children were investigated in this descriptive research. Sleep patterns, sleep disturbances, and the repercussions of disrupted sleep in school-aged children are all poorly understood. A battery of sleep questionnaires, including parent, teacher, and self-report surveys, were administered to 494 primary school students in grades kindergarten through fourth. Parent-defined sleep issues varied from 3.7 percent (Sleep-Disordered Breathing) to 15.1 percent (Bedtime Resistance), with 37 percent of the whole group having substantial sleep problems in at least one sleep category. Sleep issues were more common in younger children than in older children, as reported by parents (especially bedtime battles and night waking), teachers, and self-report. Children, as opposed to their parents, self-reported more sleep issues, notably sleep start delay and nocturnal waking. Overall, all three assessments indicated around 10% of the group as having serious issues with daytime drowsiness. The findings of this study highlight the necessity of sleep problem screening in this age range in a clinical context. It is also discussed the need for unanimity on the use of sleep screening devices and the characterization of "problem" sleep in school-aged children.[36]

Review of literature related to Sleep Assessment scale:

The study related to Pittsburgh Sleep Quality Index (PSQI) is a multidimensional sleep quality evaluation that takes into account characteristics including sleep quality, sleep latency, and sleep duration, habitual sleep efficiency, and sleep interruptions, use of sleep medications, and daytime dysfunction in the preceding month. The PSQI consists of 19 questions that you must answer and five questions that your bed partner or roommate must answer. The scale is scored only on self-reported items. The results showed that the PSQI Chinese version has convergent validity. Confirmatory factor analysis revealed that the translated PSQI data best fitted a three-component model. The ideal cut-off score for identifying insomnia was 5, which had a sensitivity of 0.81 and a specificity of 0.70. The PSQI might be used in clinical settings to evaluate early sleep disturbance. Appropriate medicines might therefore be supplied to lower long-term healthcare expenses.[37]

The study on the Pittsburgh Sleep Quality Index in Children, Adolescents, and Young Adults with Chronic Pain: Reliability, Factor Structure, and Related Clinical Factors. The Pittsburgh Sleep Quality Index (PSQI) was evaluated in a clinical sample of children, adolescents, and young adults with chronic pain for its psychometric qualities and factorial structure. Two cross-sectional studies and a chronic pain services outpatient clinic analysed a total of 482 people (aged 8 to 21). PSQI component scores were subjected to exploratory and confirmatory factor analysis, as well as reliability analysis. External validity was assessed by looking at the relationships between the PSQI global score and several clinical parameters. The results showed that a single-factor model of the PSQI is reliable and valid in a clinical sample of children with chronic pain, and they support the link between poor sleep quality and crucial clinical measures of well-being in this group. These findings support making an educated choice about its usage with this particular group and highlight the therapeutic importance of sleep quality assessment. [38]

Sleep Quality Worthy of Note in Paediatric Sleep Questionnaire for Obstructive Sleep Apnoea Syndrome Screening? On the spectrum of sleep-related respiratory problems, obstructive sleep apnoea syndrome (OSAS) is the most severe (SRBDs). Although the Paediatric Sleep Questionnaire (PSQ) is one of the most widely used and validated screening instruments, it lacks a full evaluation of several OSAS factors, such as anamnestic assessment and sleep quality. They believe that integrating characteristics that differentiate sleep quality might improve PSQ's efficiency and accuracy. [39]

The Sleep Disturbance Scale for Children (SDSC) was used in this study on babies and toddlers (6–36 months). A total of 193 healthy infants (aged 6-36 months) were examined over the course of a year using a 22-item version of the SDSC for Italian infants and toddlers. The six criteria identified reflect the most prevalent areas of sleep disturbances in children in age group, and might thus assist doctors in identifying areas that require further research. [40]

The study was conducted on development and validation of the Sleep Disturbances Scale for School-age Children. The study comprised 838 students from six primary schools, with 524 of them participating in the scale's validation procedure. This group includes children in the third through sixth grades of elementary school, with 51.1 percent of the girls and an average age of 10.3 1.3 years for the entire sample. According to statistical study, there are six significant components that account for 47.8% of total variance: 2) nightmares (= 0.76); 3) nocturnal awakenings (= 0.71); 4) daytime drowsiness (= 0.69); 5) exhaustion and trouble waking up (= 0.69); and 6) somnambulism (= 0.69). School-Age Sleep Disturbances Scale Children is a psychometrically suitable test that may be used to screen for sleep disorders in the Mexican kid population.[41]

The study shows Self-Report Subjective Sleep Measures in Children the American Academy of Sleep Medicine (AASM) has released a consensus statement on the amount of sleep that new-borns and children should have. Sleep duration, a component of sleep quality, is linked to seven health categories in children, according to the AASM expert panel. For optimal health and function, children need a certain amount of hours of sleep each night. There is a scarcity of data available to subjectively rate sleep in this group. Practitioners must assess sleep quality rather than just sleep time. ongoing research is required to develop reliable and valid self-reported sleep evaluations in children. This research is an important first step in determining the most precise subjective sleep assessments in children.[42]

Study conducted quantifying subjective assessments of sleep quality in children with enuresis, , quality of life, and depressive mood. Between the two groups, there were no significant differences in age, gender, or other demographic variables. Findings show that children with nocturnal enuresis have a substantial influence on their lives; notably as they get older, their health scores worsen, hence we recommend that therapy be started at an appropriate age according to standards.[43]

A study reported sleep disturbances in a community sample from preschool to school age. During the initial trial and the follow-up study, the parents of 481 children filled out questionnaires (girls 49 percent , boys 51 percent ; mean age 9, range 7-11). Sleep disorders decreased modestly in the population from preschool to school age (P 0.05). Sleep issues in preschool, on the other hand, lasted far into elementary school. At the follow-up, 35% of children who were diagnosed with a sleep disturbance while they were in preschool still had it at school age. This translates to about 9% of the youngsters in the neighbourhood. Children who did not have sleep issues in preschool were less likely to have sleep disorders as they became older. In paediatric health care, more emphasis should be paid to sleep issues, with therapies geared specifically at children with long-term sleep disorders.[44]

The study was conducted with the Korean version of the Pittsburgh Sleep Quality Index's reliability and validity. The Cronbach's coefficient for internal consistency of the PSQI-K total score is 0.84, indicating excellent reliability. The sensitivity and specificity for distinguishing terrible and outstanding sleepers, using the optimum cut-off value of 8.5, were 0.943 and 0.844, respectively. For insomnia and narcolepsy, the PSQI-K total and component scores were considerably higher than controls ($p < 0.05$). For the overall score, the test-retest correlation value has been 0.65 ($p < 0.001$). The two values did not vary significantly when paired t tests were used. The PSQI-K is a reliable and accurate sleep quality questionnaire for people with sleep problems. [45]

The reliability and validity of the Dutch version of the Child Sleep Habits Questionnaire were investigated in a research on sleep and sleep disruption in children. Parents returned the questionnaire in large numbers: 1502 (63 percent), 47 percent for test-retest, and 32 percent for inter observer reliability. The test-retest reliability ranged from 0.47 to 0.93, indicating moderate to high dependability. With the exception of Sleep duration, inter observer reliability was moderate to good, ranging from 0.53 to 0.87. Factor analysis reveals that the CSHQ's performance may be influenced by translation, cultural context, or subscales of the original instrument. [46]

Paediatric sleep questionnaires as diagnostic or epidemiological tools: a review of currently available instruments was the subject of an experimental investigation. An broad collection of published and unpublished instruments used to examine or evaluate sleep disorders in children was compiled and evaluated using basic instrument creation concepts (11 steps). Only a few instruments were validated and standardised using adequate psychometric criteria out of all those found. In fact, only two instruments meet all of the desired criteria, and around 11 instruments appear to meet the majority of the psychometric tool creation requirements, therefore they were given a closer look. Paediatric sleep questionnaires as diagnostic or epidemiological tools: a review of currently available instruments was the subject of an experimental investigation. An broad collection of published and unpublished instruments used to examine or evaluate sleep disorders in children was compiled and evaluated using basic instrument creation concepts (11 steps). Only a few instruments were validated and standardised using adequate psychometric criteria out of all those found. In fact, only two instruments meet all of the desired criteria, and around 11 instruments appear to meet the majority of the psychometric tool creation requirements, therefore they were given a closer look.[47]

A study conducted by researcher in children with monosymptomatic nocturnal enuresis, researchers looked at probable declines in QoL and sleep quality, as well as the relationship among these variables. The study included 44 children with mono symptomatic nocturnal enuresis and 27 healthy controls ranging in age from 6 to 15.[39]

Translation, cultural modification, and validation of a sleep disruption measure for children. In order to validate semantic, experiential, conceptual, and cultural equivalence, the scale instructions and items were standardized. The visual communication scale structure was also customised to the preferences and habits of the Brazilian people, resulting in a chart with clear instructions and simple recognition of the statements and alternative replies. Values larger than 0.55 were found in the reliability analysis. There has been convergent validity that is credible. The PSG study found that discriminating validity for positive sleep-disordered breathing (SDB) was 8.9, indicating that discriminatory validity was only tested for SDB. The scale's three questions can be used to screen for SDB. Internal consistency, convergent and discriminatory validity, and internal consistency were all present in the SDSC after it was translated, Standardized, and validated into Brazilian Portuguese. It can be used to screen for sleep-disordered breathing in children in population-based investigations. [48]

The current study assessed the Children's Sleep Habits Questionnaire in toddlers and preschool children. The CSHQ in a younger age range and a more varied population than previously reported. A total of 194 children, ranging in age from 2 to 512 years, were divided into three diagnostic groups: 68 children with autism, 57 children with developmental delay without autism, and 69 children who were typically developing. All parents completed the CSHQ and a sleep record, and all children were subjected to actigraphy for seven days and nights. On the basis of a parent report of a general sleep issue at the time of enrolment into the research, the children were split into problem sleep and non-problem sleep groups. The issue and non-problem sleep groups' CSHQ results were then compared. The findings imply that the CSHQ is therapeutically relevant for detecting sleep disorders in normally developing infants as well as children with a variety of neurodevelopment abnormalities at these young ages. The somewhat higher subscale ratings in younger children than previously reported for older children appear to be associated with more sleep issues. [49]

The cohort study related Children Sleep Habits Questionnaire (CSHQ): psychometric validation in Indian school children. The average score for the study was 49.35. (S.D. 7.6). CSHQ scale items showed acceptable overall internal consistency (Cronbach's alpha 0.77), but its subscales were unreliable. Excluding the youngest school children (class Pre-Nursery) from the data analysis considerably increased the internal consistency alphas of the various subscales, demonstrating that CSHQ subscales are more reliable in later age groups in our environment. CSHQ exhibited strong concurrent validity when compared to the Visual Analogue Scale (VAS) for global sleep assessment. Construct validity of CSHQ was evaluated by principal factor analysis which extracted 8 underlying latent factors (with Eigen value >1) matching original CSHQ domains. However, these latent factors explained only 48.2% of total variance in the data. Principal Component Analysis (PCA) of CSHQ in our study cohort also favours shortening of original 33-item scale to a shorter 23-item scale with better acceptability for parents. The CSHQ is a reliable and internally consistent scale, and it is useful optional tool for assessing sleep problems in Indian school children. [50]

The study was conducted at community-based paediatric clinic and a university-affiliated hospital A total of 108 S-SDB patients (mean [standard deviation] age: 7 +/- 4 years) and 72 healthy controls (8 +/- 4 years) were enlisted. The Conners Abbreviated Symptom Questionnaire and a Standardized Epworth Sleepiness Scale (ESS) were used. Patients with S-SDB underwent polysomnography. In comparison to control participants, patients with S-SDB had a higher ESS (8.1 +/- 4.9 vs 5.3 +/- 3.9) and a higher Conners score (12.8 +/- 7.6 vs 9.0 +/- 6.2). EDS was diagnosed in 28% of individuals based on adult criteria. Patients with primary snoring and those with obstructive sleep apnea had similar ESS and Conners scores. The ESS and polysomnographic parameters exhibited modest relationships. Children with S-SDB were sleepier and hyperactive than control participants, while possessing an ESS score that was within the normal range for adults. However, a population-based investigation should corroborate this findings.[51]

The study related to the paediatric daytime sleepiness scale (PDSS): “sleep habits and school outcomes in middle-school children. Factor analysis on the 13 questions related to daytime sleepiness yielded 1 primary factor ("paediatric daytime sleepiness"; 32% of variance). Only items with factor loadings above .4 were included in the final sleepiness scale. Internal consistency (Chronbach's alpha) for the final 8-item scale was .80. Separate one-way analyses of variance and trend analyses were performed comparing paediatric daytime sleepiness scores at the 5 different levels of total sleep time and academic achievement. Participants who reported low school achievement, high rates of absenteeism, low school enjoyment, low total sleep time, and frequent illness reported significantly higher levels of daytime sleepiness compared to children with better school-related outcomes. The self-report scale developed in the present work is suitable for middle-school-age children and may be useful in future research given its ease of administration and robust psychometric properties. Daytime sleepiness is related to reduce educational achievement and other negative school-related outcomes”.[52]

The test-retest reliability and validity of the Pittsburgh Sleep Quality Index in primary insomnia were reported in a study. In primary insomnia patients, the overall PSQI global score correlation coefficient for test-retest reliability was.87. Validity studies found strong links between the PSQI and sleep log data, but not so much with polysomnography data. As a predictor of sleep disruptions in insomnia patient's vs controls, a PSQI global score > 5 had a sensitivity of 98.7 and specificity of 84.4. For patients with primary insomnia, the PSQI has high test-retest reliability and validity. [53]

A study conducted validity and reliability of scales for sleep-disordered breathing, snoring, drowsiness, and behavioural disorders were investigated by a researcher using the paediatric sleep questionnaire (PSQ). Based on data from a randomly selected 50% of the individuals (group A), item reduction yielded a 22-item SRBD score that was substantially linked with diagnosis of an SRBD (P0.0001) in a logistic regression model that took age and gender into account. Among group A patients, diagnosis was also substantially linked to sub-scores for snoring (four items, P0.0001), tiredness (four items, P=0.0003), and behaviour (six items, P0.0001). The scales performed comparably well in both group B and group C individuals, as well as in people of various ages and genders. A selected criteria SRBD score yielded a sensitivity of 0.85 and 0.81 in group A and B participants, respectively; a specificity of 0.87 and 0.87 in group B individuals; and a proper classification for 86 and 85 percent of subjects. The scales have strong internal consistency and test-retest stability in a different sample (n=21).[54]

The Children's Sleep Disturbance Scale (SDSC) Construction and validation of a sleep disturbances assessment tool for children and adolescents. To attempt a categorization of sleep disorders in children, we developed a 27 item Likert-type rating scale (Sleep Disturbance Scale for Children: SDSC) and assessed the psychometric properties was developed.

The scale was given out to 1304 moms with children (1157 controls, mean age 9.8 y; 147 sleep disorder subjects, mean age 9.2y, composed of four clinical groups: Insomnia 39 subjects, Hypersomnia 12 subjects, Respiratory disturbances during sleep 25 subjects and Parasomnias 71 subjects). Internal consistency was excellent in controls (0.79) and remained good in sleep problem patients (0.71); test/retest reliability was adequate for both total and single item scores (r = 0.71). The component analysis revealed six variables that characterised the most prevalent regions of sleep disturbances in infancy and adolescence (variance explained 44.21 percent). Enuresis was the sole item with a factor loading less than 0.40 and a poor inter-item correlation, thus it was dropped from the final scale, leaving a total of 26 items. The validity and discriminating power of the measures between controls and the four clinical groups were validated by a re-evaluation of the sample using factor scores. The notion that childhood sleep disorders are not independent entities or cluster into multiple groups connected to each other was confirmed by the association between factor scores. In both clinical and non-clinical groups, the SDSC appears to be an effective tool for assessing sleep disorders in school-aged children.[55]

Abstracts from Meta-analysis and Systemic reviews

A meta-analysis and comprehensive investigation of the incidence of sleep difficulties among children in mainland China. This meta-analysis included 66 papers, revealing that the pooled prevalence of sleep difficulties was 37.6 percent (95 percent CI: 34.3-40.9 percent) with substantial heterogeneity (I2 = 99.6 percent, P 0.001). Snoring was 7.7%, choking or gasping was 0.9 percent, apnea was 1.5 percent, restless sleep was 11.3 percent, mouth breathing was 4.7 percent, hyperhidrosis was 17.2%, leg movements were 2.7 percent, bruxism was 9.6%, sleep talking was 0.7 percent, sleep-walking was 0.8 percent, nightmare was 5.1 percent, enuresis was 3.4 percent, night awakening was 6.7 percent, and trouble falling asleep was 11.1 Males had a greater prevalence rate of sleep difficulties than females (OR:1.01,95 percent CI:1.05-1.13). The incidence of sleep disorders rose with age in all age categories, including infancy or early childhood (33.3 percent), pre-school (38.9%), and school-age (43.7 percent). South China had the lowest prevalence rate (30.4 percent, 95 percent CI: 23.9-36.8%), while West China had the greatest prevalence rate (47.4 percent, 95 percent CI: 35.9-58.9%), which was higher than any other area in China. The CSHQ criterion yielded a higher point estimate for sleep disorders prevalence than other criteria. The age group might impact prevalence estimate, according to meta-regression (P = 0.011). Sleep disorders have been more common among youngsters in mainland China over the last two decades, impacting about one-fifth of school-aged children. Hyperhidrosis, restless sleep, and difficulty falling asleep were all more common than other sleep problems. West China has a much greater incidence of sleep difficulties than any other region. Because there are currently no recommendations on children's sleep difficulties in mainland China, future study should focus on school-aged children and children from economically disadvantaged regions.[56]

A comprehensive study and meta-analysis found that passive body heating in the form of a warm shower or bath before night improves sleep: Before night, water-based passive body heating (PBHWB) in the form of a warm shower or bath is frequently advised as an easy way to improve sleep. To investigate the effects of PBHWB on sleep onset latency (SOL), wake after sleep onset, total sleep time, sleep efficiency (SE), slow wave sleep, and subjective sleep quality, the researcher searched PubMed, CINAHL, Cochran, Medline, PsycInfo, and Web of Science databases and extracted pertinent information from publications meeting predefined inclusion and exclusion criteria. After deleting duplicates, the search revealed 5322 candidate papers, 17 of which matched the inclusion requirements and 13 of which provided comparable quantitative data for meta-analyses. PBHWB of 40-42.5 °C was related with better self-rated sleep quality and SE, as well as considerable reduction of SOL when scheduled 1-2 hours before bedtime for as little as 10 minutes. The level of core body temperature fall obtained by enhanced blood circulation to the palms and soles augments the distal-to-proximal skin temperature gradient to boost body heat dissipation, according to these findings. Nonetheless, further study is needed because the findings on PBHWB are restricted by the relative lack of published research, particularly on its ideal timing and duration, as well as specific mechanisms of benefits.[57]

Review of literature related to BEARS scale

The study was conducted to assess individuals with mono symptomatic enuresis, sleep hygiene and the incidence of sleep disorders. The average age is 9.7 ±3.0 years. Age, gender, BMI, tonsillectomy history, asthma, and sleep time hours had no statistically significant differences. Patients with MEN had a greater proportion of abnormalities in their sleep hygiene than controls. The BEARS questionnaire revealed that patients with MEN had a greater prevalence of sleep disturbances than the other two groups: 60.7 percent (n=74) vs 18.6 percent (n=32) and 38.3 percent (n=18) for controls and ANTENUR, respectively ($p<.05$). Sleep disruptions and sleep disorders were more common in MEN children than with controls. The BEARS questionnaire is an effective clinical tool for detecting sleep disturbances in kids.[58]

The BEARS sleep disorder questionnaire's reliability and validity in children and adolescents from Bogotá, Colombia. Sleep is critical for school-aged children's health and well-being. The purpose of this study was to examine the BEARS questionnaire's reliability and content validity in children and adolescents aged 9 to 17. In Bogotá, Colombia, the poll included 8,862 children and adolescents from 24 recognised educational institutions. Participants were given the BEARS questionnaire in a structured, self-administered format. A sub-sample of 246 people was used to conduct reliability tests. The consistency, construct validity, and reliability of the instrument were assessed using Cronbach's alpha coefficient, exploratory factor analysis (EFA), and the weighted Kappa coefficient. The findings showed acceptable consistency and reliability (global Cronbach's alpha = 0.732; range = 0.706 to 0.769). (Kappa = 0.665; range = 0.706–0.769) The EFA found a single factor (item 1: sleep troubles) that explained 61.4 percent of the variance by combining two interactions 2/gl = 2690.817; p = 0.001. The BEARS questionnaire's internal consistency, reliability, and validity were all good. As a result of these results, this instrument is largely recommended for use in primary care in Bogotá, Colombia, for investigating and screening sleep disorders in school-aged populations.[59]

A study was conducted on Sleep hygiene behaviours and patterns among Nigerian school-aged adolescents. 61.8 percent of the 353 adolescents tested were boys, while 38.2 percent were girls, for a male-to-female ratio of 1.6:1. Early, middle, and late teens made up 13.9 percent, 39.9%, and 46.2 percent of the total, respectively. The most prevalent sleep-related concern indicated by BEARS sleep screening participants was nocturnal awakenings (34.6 percent), followed by excessive daytime tiredness (21.0 percent). Sleep duration was 7.19 1.26, 7.13 1.13, and 7.16 1.28 years old, with P > 0.05. Although 62.9 percent of all teenagers watched TV/played video games until one-hour prior bedtime, it was not statistically linked to any of the sleep disorders, with the highest prevalence in late adolescence. In Kano, Nigerian teenagers' sleep quality and quantity are both inadequate. Our society should pay greater attention to adolescent and sleep medicine. [60]

The study conducted on Rural Preschool Aged Children's Sleep Problems .A total of 80 preschoolers were investigated. The majority of the youngsters (37.50 percent) were between the ages of 49 and 60 months. 45 children (56.25%) needed bedtime patting. Sleep talking and nocturnal enuresis affected 20 (25%) of the youngsters. On the BEARS test, the majority of children

(23.7%) experienced bedtime issues, whereas only 6.5% had sleep disordered breathing. Joint family (2 = 12.58, df = 1, p = 0.0004, HS) and working parents had more specific sleep issues. Sleep disturbances in rural preschool children has prevalent and clinically significant. Examining sleep in children should be as natural and routine for doctors as examining food, exercise, and development.[61]

A first evaluation of the BEARS sleep screening tool for children in Spanish for concurrent validity. In this cross-sectional descriptive research, a registered nurse used the BEARS to a sample of 60 parents of children aged 2–16 years (n = 60, 71.7 percent male) who attended a mental healthcare institution (located in Murcia, Spain) for the first time to receive a group psycho educational intervention. Mann–Whitney The association between the information obtained with the BEARS and scores on the CSHQ's corresponding subscales was investigated using U tests. Children with a sleep issue, according to the BEARS, scored substantially higher on the CSHQ-related subscales than children without a sleep problem (all Ps <0.05). Our findings confirm the BEARS Spanish translation's concurrent validity in detecting sleep issues in paediatric nursing evaluations. More research with larger and more diverse samples is required. [62]

J Preschool Children in Qazvin, Iran, Have Sleep Issues. With an average age of 4.1 years, the research population included 299 boys (51.6%) and 280 girls (48.3%) (SD 0.8). The average body mass index (BMI) of the youngsters was 15. (SD 2.1). Every day, the children slept for an average of 10:54 hours (SD 00:48). They went to bed early (23:18 h) and awakened late (SD 00:48). (09:26 h; SD 01:00). 6.9% of the participants claimed they were drowsy most of the time. Sleep-disordered breathing, snoring, and waking up in the middle of the night were all recorded at 13.9 percent, 1.2 percent, and 2.7 percent, respectively. The majority of the kids (87%) slept in the same room as their parents (P > 0.05). The children had late bedtimes, delayed sleep onset, daytime sleepiness, nightly awakenings, sleep-disordered breathing, and snoring. Iranian teenagers have a reputation for sharing rooms.[63]

Bharti B, etA guide for primary care physicians who treat children with sleep issues. Sleep difficulties are common in children, affecting 20–42 percent of them. A sleep problem is often characterised as an insufficient sleeping pattern that generates concern in the parent, kid, or physician. Children see primary care doctors or paediatricians for three forms of sleep problems: dyssomnias, hypersomnias, and parasomnias. When examining a child with a sleep problem, a detailed sleep history is followed by a complete medical, developmental, and behavioural history. BEARS (B is for bedtime difficulties, E is for excessive daytime drowsiness, A is for nightly awakenings, R is for regularity as well as duration of sleep, and S is for snoring) is a simple sleep screening tool for children. This article discusses common sleep issues in children of all ages, from infancy through puberty, as well as therapy options for improving children's sleep outcomes.[64]

A study related to population-based research found a high frequency of sleep difficulties among school-aged and preschool-aged children in Tehran. The BEARS questionnaire was completed by 746 children aged 2 to 12: 325 in pre-school (2-6 years old) (142 females [43.7 percent] and 183 boys [56.3 percent]) and 421 in primary school (7-12 years old), with average ages of 3.93 (±0.16) and 9.63 (±0.16) years, respectively. Excessive daytime drowsiness was the most prevalent screening issue in both groups (64.9 percent and 62.9 percent respectively). In the pre-school age group, bedtime issues, as well as sleep regularity and duration, were substantially higher (P0.0002; odds ratio [OR] =1.98; 95 percent confidence interval [95 percent CI]: 1.98-4.20; and OR=2.00; 95 percent CI: 1.41- 2.84, respectively). The difference in mean sleep duration between pre-school and school-age groups was statistically significant (P0.0001). According to the present study, various forms of sleep difficulties are rather common among preschool and school-aged children, especially when it comes to excessive afternoon sleeping. Within the pre-school age group, bedtime and regularity issues were substantially more prominent. School entry seems to be beneficial for bedtime issues and sleep-disordered breathing. [65]

A study was cited regarding sleeping patterns of Iranian pre-school children in a city: Children's sleep debt and late sleeping with 224 participants, according to screening tools such as the BEARS and CSHQ (Children's Sleep Habits Questionnaires), Iranian children had shorter night sleep duration than expected for their age group (9.54 vs 12 h). Earlier sleepers had greater total daily sleep time (11:36 1:42; 10:36 1:30 h, P = 0.005) and night sleep duration (10:36 1:12; 9:12 1:06 h, P > 0.001). The bulk of nappers (85 percent) gone to bed around 22:00 or later. Iranian preschool children's poor sleep quality is most likely attributable to cultural differences, climatic variances, or hazardous sleep practises. [66]

BEARS is a sleeping evaluation tool. The BEARS is a five-item screening instrument for children who are in basic care. Each letter of the test's acronym indicates one of the five issues to explore, making the instrument "user-friendly" for families and easy to remember for doctors: Bedtime difficulties, excessive daytime weariness, nocturnal awakenings, sleep regularity and duration, and snoring are all factors to consider. Parents are asked whether they have any concerns in each area, and if they do, physicians will ask for extra information (e.g., frequency and kind of problem) (e.g., frequency and nature of problem).[67]

A study was conducted on sleep issues in rural Indian preschool and school-aged youngsters. They examined 513 children (2–6 years old = 252; 7–12 years old = 261) who came to a rural medical college hospital's paediatric outpatient for sleep problems using the 'BEARS' approach. Sleep problems identified in the BEARS domains for preschool (2–6 years, P=0.1) included bedtime problems (33.3 percent vs 14.9 percent, P0.001), excessive daytime sleepiness (32.5 percent vs 1.9 percent, P0.001), awakening during the night (25 percent vs 11.87 percent, P0.001), regularity and duration of sleep (19.84 percent vs 4.98 percent, P0.001), and sleep disordered breathing (4.8 percent vs 5 percent, P= Sleep problems are common among rural Indian children, and they should be checked for at routine medical visits.[68]

The Persian version of the "BEARS" paediatric sleep questionnaire has tested for reliability and validity. To test the reliability and validity of the Persian version of the "BEARS" paediatric sleep questionnaire. Two paediatric primary care clinics in Tehran, Iran. BEARS sleep questionnaire was performed in the first stage, and then BEARS was done again (by another questioner) and all of the individuals were seen by sleep experts for diagnosis of sleep problems. BEARS results were compared across time and amongst various questioners to establish test-retest reliability. BEARS data were matched to expert diagnoses to assess criterion validity. The study included 215 children aged 2 to 12 years old. There were 101 preschoolers (2-6 years old) and 114 primary school students among them (7-12 years old). All BEARS items in the preschool age group and the majority of items in the school age group had high to excellent test-retest reliability (P0.05). In both age groups, almost half of the items were legitimate (P0.05). The application of BEARS (a basic brief screening instrument for paediatric sleep issues) in children, particularly in Persian, seems to be a trustworthy and somewhat valid sleep screening technique.[69]

A pilot study of the use of the 'BEARS' sleep assessment instrument in a paediatric residents' continuity clinic. The BEARS (B=Bedtime Issues, E=Excessive Daytime Sleepiness, A=Night Awakenings, R=Regularity and Duration of Sleep, S=Snoring) was developed to see how successful a basic 5-item paediatric sleep screening tool is in gathering sleep-related data and detecting sleep issues in primary care settings. In a tertiary care children's hospital, paediatric residents have a continuity clinic. During the 5-month trial period, BEARS forms were included into the medical files of a sample consisting of 2 to 12 year old children who were seeing their paediatrician for a well-child exam. Sleep-related data from the BEARS visit and the pre-BEARS appointment, which would have been the subject's most recent previous well child check (WCC), were coded to see whether a sleep issue existed and if it had been corrected. Pre-BEARS and BEARS WCC visits were documented for a total of 195 children. BEARS visits were significantly more likely than pre-BEARS visits to record any sleep information (98.5 percent vs. 87.7%, p0.001), as well as information about bedtime issues (93.3 percent vs. 7.7%, p0.001), excessive daytime sleepiness (93.9 percent vs. 5.6 percent, p0.001), snoring (92.8 percent vs. 7.2 percent, p0.001), and nighttimes awakenings (91.3 percent vs. 29Significantly more sleep issues were seen during the BEARS sessions in the areas of bedtime worries (16.3 percent vs. 4.1 percent, p0.001), overnight awakenings (18.4 percent vs. 6.8 percent, p0.001), and snoring (10.7 percent vs. 4.6 percent, p=0.012). Finally, sleep was mentioned in almost twice as many BEARS charts (13.1 percent vs. 7.3 percent), indicating a statistically significant difference (p=0.07). The BEARS seems to be a user-friendly paediatric sleep screening tool that significantly increases the amount of sleep data collected and the likelihood of finding sleep problems in primary care.[70]

A study was carried out to determine the subjective sleep quality of people with iron deficient anemia. According to the HAD scale, patients had an average anxiety level of 9.244.37, whereas controls had an average anxiety score of 7.58.07. In addition, the average depression score in patients was 7.534.10, whereas it was 6.412.74 in controls. Patients had a total sleep quality score of 6.713.02, whereas controls had a score of 4.111.64. In terms of anxiety, depression, and sleep quality, there was a statistically significant difference. There was no link between anxiety and depression and poor sleeping habits, according to linear regression analysis. IDA has an effect on sleep quality regardless of psychological conditions like sadness or anxiety. [71]

The study reported that Children with neuro-developmental disorders have sleep abnormalities and patterns. In these populations, we discovered variations in sleep disruptions and sleep diary metrics based on age, diagnosis, and medication usage. High nighttime waking duration was linked to sensory circumstances. The most prevalent complaint from parents was that their child's sleep was too short. Long-term concerns for parental presence at night for sleep anxiety, melatonin usage and effectiveness, and consideration for therapies to minimize daytime weariness in children aged 7–11 years old are all highlighted as key issues for additional study[72]

Narasimhan U, Anitha FS, Anbu C. (2020) The spectrum of sleep disorders among children: a cross-sectional study at a South Indian tertiary care hospital. Between November 2018 and June 2019, 450 children visited the paediatric outpatient department of Sri Ramachandra Institute of Higher Education and Research in Chennai, India for this cross-sectional research. Children with chronic diseases or a recent history of physical or emotional stress were excluded from the study. The Sleep Disturbance Scale for Children (SDSC) was developed to collect data on sleep disturbances in children. The bulk of the individuals (72.2 percent) slept 9-11 hours every day, according to the findings. The time difference between bedtime and sleep time was less than 15 minutes for 46.2 percent of the subjects. In all, 34% of the individuals reported having sleep issues. Sleep issues as a youngster, the lack of siblings, and parental presence while sleeping were all shown to be statistically significant risk factors for childhood sleep disorders (p:0.05).[73]

Merz EL, Tomfohr-Madsen L. (2018) Sleep disruption in paediatric cancer survivors: Conceptual framework and opportunities for clinical assessment and behavioural treatment. In both juvenile patients and survivors, sleep disturbance is a typical side effect of cancer and its therapy. This article reviews typical sleep issues in this demographic and offers a multidimensional framework of children cancer-specific risk factors that may combine to cause and perpetuate sleep disruption. Based on the available literature, the most important risk factors for sleep disruption in this population are cancer and its treatment parameters, physical and social environmental conditions both during and after treatment, changes in family behaviour and norms, psychological factors and traumatic stress, and reduced physical activity. Potential clinical assessment methodologies and behavioural treatments relevant to these difficulties are described with reference to the behavioural model of insomnia. The review concludes with recommendations for future research and clinical practise, including the development and testing of comprehensive assessment tools, intervention effectiveness studies in both oncology and primary care clinics, and efforts in paediatric oncology to improve sleep communication between patients and providers.[74]

Rabner J, etal (2017) Paediatric headache and sleep disturbance: a comparison of diagnostic groups. "Sleep disturbance was greater in patients with TTH ($10.34 \pm 5.94, P = .002$) and NDPH ($11.52 \pm 6.40, P < .001$) than migraine (8.31 ± 5.89). Across patient groups, greater sleep disturbance was significantly associated with higher levels of functional disability ($rs \geq .16$), anxiety ($rs \geq .30$), and depression ($rs \geq .32$). Additionally, higher pain levels were significantly associated with greater sleep disturbance among TTH patients ($r = .23$), with this association non-significant among the other headache groups. When simultaneously examining demographic, pain-related, and emotional distress factors, older age, higher levels of disability and depression, and NDPH diagnosis were all significant predictors of greater sleep disturbance ($r^2 = .25$).Assessment and treatment of sleep problems in pediatric patients with chronic headache is important with several contextual and headache diagnostic factors influencing the severity of sleep disturbance".[75]

Hale L, Guan S. (2015) A thorough literature evaluation of screen time and sleep among school-aged children and adolescents. The scientific literature on the relationship between screen time (e.g., television, computers, video games, and mobile devices) and sleep outcomes in school-aged children and adolescents was comprehensively reviewed and updated. We looked at 67 papers that were published between 1999 and early 2014. In 90 percent of research, we discovered that screen time is negatively connected with sleep outcomes (mainly reduced length and delayed timing). The results varied depending on the type of screen exposure, the participant's age, gender, and the day of the week. While the evidence for a link between screen time and sleep is strong, there are some limitations to the existing research: 1.) there is no proof of a causative relationship; 2.) there is measurement error (in both screen time exposure and sleep measurements); 3.) there is a lack of data on simultaneous usage of many screens, as well as the features and content of the screens utilized. To avoid any negative impacts of screen time on sleep and well-being, youth should be counseled to restrict or reduce screen time exposure, particularly before or during bedtime hours. Future study should take into account the methodological constraints of existing studies, as well as the size and mechanisms of the connection. These stages will aid in the creation and execution of policies or interventions aimed at reducing youth screen time. [76]

Lewandowski AS, Ward TM, Palermo TM. (2011) Children and teenagers with common medical illnesses have sleep issues. Children's health and well-being are dependent on their ability to sleep. Sleep disruptions and disorders that go untreated can have serious implications during the day and put children at risk for ill health. When compared to their generally healthy counterparts, children with acute and chronic medical illnesses have more sleep disruptions. Sleep disturbances in medically ill children can be associated with sleep disorders (e.g., sleep disordered breathing, restless leg syndrome), co-morbid with acute and chronic conditions (e.g., asthma, arthritis, cancer), or secondary to underlying disease-related mechanisms (e.g. airway restriction, inflammation) treatment regimens, or hospitalization. Clinical management should include a multidisciplinary approach with particular emphasis on routine, regular sleep assessments and prevention of daytime consequences and promotion of healthy sleep habits and health outcomes. [77]

Heyer GL, etal (2014). Specific headache factors predict sleep disturbances among youth with migraine. "Fifty-two patients generated 4680 diary entries, 984 patients (21%) involved headaches. Headache intensity ($P = 0.009$) and timing of headache onset ($P < 0.001$) were predictive of sleep disturbances. Three Paediatric Migraine Disability Assessment-based items were also associated with sleep disturbances: partial school-day absence ($P = 0.04$), recreational activities prevented ($P < 0.001$), and decreased functioning during recreational activities ($P < 0.001$). Sleep disturbances correlated positively and significantly with daily headache disability scores ($r_{pb} = 0.35$; $P < 0.01$).We conclude that specific headache factors predict sleep disturbances among youth with primary headaches". [78]

Orsey AD, Wakefield DB, Cloutier MM. (2013) "Physical activity (PA) and sleep among children and adolescents with cancer. Participants had impaired sleep based upon normative data compiled from multiple studies of more than 1,700 healthy children from 1 to 18 years of age, including decreased total sleep time (mean 6.6 hours, standard deviation (SD) 1.3 hours), increased wake after sleep onset (WASO; mean 2 hours, SD 1.4 hours), increased awakenings during sleep (mean 28.3 wake bouts, SD 7.8 bouts), and decreased sleep efficiency (mean 74.2%, SD 13.3%). Fatigue correlated with self-reported sleep quality but not with disturbances in sleep as measured by actigraphy. In longitudinal models that controlled for age, diagnosis group, gender, race, and steroid use, higher average activity, as measured by actigraphy, was associated with improved sleep quantity (P = 0.005) and efficiency (P = 0.001).Paediatric oncology patients demonstrate impaired sleep. Greater PA was significantly associated with improved sleep quantity and efficiency in paediatric oncology participants. As a potentially modifiable factor, PA may offer a mechanism to improve sleep in paediatric oncology patients". [79]

Dosi C, etal (2013) "Co morbidities of sleep disorders in childhood and adolescence: focus on migraine. The correlation and/or co morbidity between sleep disorders and headache has been reported in numerous studies, but the exact nature of the association between headache, disordered sleep, and underlying mechanisms remains poorly understood. The bidirectional association between sleep and headache is mediated by a temporal link (headache occurs during sleep, after sleep, and in relationship with sleep stages), by a quantitative relationship (excess, lack, bad quality, short duration of sleep may trigger headache), and by a reciprocal connection (headache may cause sleep disruption and may be associated with several sleep disturbances). This association is most evident for primary headache disorders, especially in childhood". A congenital alteration of neurotransmitter pathways (serotoninergic and dopaminergic) might predispose individuals to both disorders, presenting as sleep–wake rhythm disorder in infancy or as headache disorder later in childhood, as result of this neurotransmitter imbalance. Clinicians should be aware that a complete clinical evaluation of childhood headache includes a careful sleep history, taking into account that the treatment of sleep disturbances could lead to an improvement of headache symptoms and vice versa". [80]

Alfano CA, Kim KL. (2011) "Objective sleep patterns and severity of symptoms in paediatric obsessive compulsive disorder: a pilot investigation. Sleep disturbances are common among youth with anxiety disorders, yet objective assessments of sleep in children with obsessive compulsive disorder (OCD) have been the focus of scant research. We therefore compared a small group of non-medicated, non-depressed children with primary OCD (ages 7-11 years) to matched healthy controls using home-based actigraphy during a 7-day prospective assessment. Validated parent and child sleep measures also were collected, and associations among objective sleep variables and severity of obsessions and compulsions were examined. We found significantly fragmented sleep patterns in the OCD group compared to controls including reduced total sleep time (TST) and longer wake periods after sleep onset. Severity of compulsions showed a significant negative correlation with TST. These preliminary findings indicate the presence of sleep abnormalities in pre-pubescent OCD patients with potential implications for future examinations of early developmental processes and features of the disorder". [81]

Bell JF, Zimmerman FJ. (2010) "Shortened night-time sleep duration in early life and subsequent childhood obesity. For younger children (aged 0-4 years at baseline), short duration of night-time sleep at baseline was strongly associated with increased risk of subsequent overweight or obesity (odds ratio = 1.80; 95% confidence interval, 1.16-2.80). For older children (aged 5-13 years), baseline sleep was not associated with subsequent weight status; however, contemporaneous sleep was inversely associated. Daytime sleep had little effect on subsequent obesity in either group. Shortened sleep duration in early life is a modifiable risk factor with important implications for obesity prevention and treatment. Insufficient night time sleep among infants and preschool-aged children may be a lasting risk factor for subsequent obesity. Napping does not appear to be a substitute for night time sleep in terms of obesity prevention". [82]

Hysing M, etal (2009) Sleep in children with chronic illness, and the relation to emotional and behavioural problems—a population-based study. There were no differences in time in bed between children with a chronic illness and their healthy peers. However, the chronic illness group reported more problems falling asleep and had more night time awakenings. The increased risk for sleep problems was reduced to a non significant level when adjusting for emotional and behavioural problems. The elevated rate of sleep problems and association with emotional and behavioural problems in children with chronic illness underline the importance of early detection and intervention in this group. [84]

Sivertsen B, etal (2009) "Chronicity of sleep problems in children with chronic illness: a longitudinal population-based study. 295 of 4025 (7.3%) children had a chronic illness, and the prevalence of chronic sleep problems was significantly higher in this group compared to children without chronic illness (6.8% versus 3.6%). Sleep problems at the first wave increased the risk of sleep problems at the second wave, also when adjusting for potential confounders (odds-ratio = 5.41). Hyperactivity and emotional problems were also independent risk factors for later sleep problems. These findings call for increased awareness and development of treatment strategies of sleep problems in children with chronic illness". [85]

Stores G. (2009) "Aspects of sleep disorders in children and adolescents. Sleep disorders in children and adolescents is a topic that has been, and remains, neglected in both public health education and professional training. Although much knowledge has been accumulated in recent times, it has been poorly disseminated and, therefore, relatively little is put into practice. Only some general issues can be discussed in this article. The aspects chosen relate mainly to clinical practice, but they also have relevance for research. They concern various differences between sleep disorders in children and those in adults, the occurrence of such disorders in young people, their effects on psychological and physical development, the essential (but often ignored) distinction between sleep problems and their underlying causes (ie, sleep disorders), types of sleep disturbance encountered at different ages during development, and the differential diagnosis of certain parasomnias that are at particular risk of being confused with each other". [86]

Long AC, Krishnamurthy V, Palermo TM. (2008) "Sleep disturbances in school-age children with chronic pain. Levels of overall sleep disturbances were above the clinical cutoff for 53% of children with chronic pain. Sleep disturbances predicted lower physical HRQOL and higher functional disability, according to parent report. Sleep disturbances are common and associated with daytime functioning in school-age children with chronic pain, suggesting that assessment and treatment of sleep problems is clinically relevant". [87]

Hart CN, Jelalian E. (2008) "Shortened sleep duration is associated with paediatric overweight. Increasing attention is being focused on potential risk factors that may lead to overweight in children and adolescents and that may, therefore, be important targets for intervention. Historically, children's eating and activity habits have received considerable attention in programmatic research targeted at prevention and treatment of overweight. However, more recent research has found that additional factors may play a role in this growing epidemic. Of particular interest is children's sleep duration. The goal of this article is to review research that has assessed the association between children's sleep duration and overweight risk in an attempt to uncover the potential role of sleep in the growing obesity epidemic. Although shortened sleep duration is associated with increased overweight in children, additional research is needed prior to recommending that children's sleep be increased as a means to address the current obesity epidemic". [88]

Isik U, etal (2007). "Prevalence of headache and its association with sleep disorders in children. An association between headache and sleep disturbances has been reported in previous studies, but there is a lack of research examining this relationship in a community sample of children in order to reveal the magnitude of the problem. Among 32 District Educational Directorates in Istanbul, nine school districts and within each district eight schools were randomly selected. A questionnaire consisting of socio demographic variables and evaluating headache and sleep disturbances was sent to students' homes to be completed by their parents. The prevalence of headache was 31.4% (95% confidence interval: 29.5-33.4%). Migraine prevalence was 3.3%, whereas no migraine headache prevalence was 28.1%. The prevalence of headache was similar between males and females (29.6% vs 33.3%, $P > 0.05$). The frequency of headache increased with age for both sexes. Snoring, parasomnias, sweating during sleep, and day time sleepiness were more common among children with migraine compared with no migraine and no headache groups. Headaches are common among schoolchildren. Because children with migraine headaches have a high prevalence of sleep disturbances, they should always be evaluated for the presence of sleep problems". [89]

Fricke-OerkermannL,etal (2007). "Prevalence and course of sleep problems in childhood. Children and parents were surveyed using questionnaires 3 times on an annual basis. In self- and parental reports, about 30%-40% of the children of the longitudinal sample had problems falling asleep at the first assessment. One year later, about 30% to 40% of these children did not describe any difficulties initiating sleep, whereas about 60% did report continuing difficulties initiating sleep. Difficulties maintaining sleep are less common in childhood. The analysis of self- and parental reports revealed that in general children described significantly more difficulties initiating and maintaining sleep than their parents report. Difficulties initiating and maintaining sleep may be transient or persistent. In practice, children and adolescents should be included in the diagnostic and therapeutic process". [90]

Smaldone A, Honig JC, Byrne MW. (2007) "Sleepless in America: inadequate sleep and relationships to health and well-being of our nation's children. Parents of elementary school-aged children with inadequate sleep were more likely to report that their child was having problems at school or had a father with fair or poor health. Parents of adolescents with inadequate sleep were more likely to report that their child had an atopic condition, frequent or severe headaches, a parent with less-than-excellent emotional health, or experienced frequent parental anger. Inadequate sleep in both age groups was associated with parental report that their child usually or always displayed depressive symptomatology, family disagreements involved heated arguing, or parental concern that the child was not always safe at home, at school, or in their neighbourhood. Approximately 15 million American children are affected by inadequate sleep. Primary care providers should routinely identify and address inadequate sleep and its associated health, school, and family factors". [91]

Russo PM, etal (2007) Sleep habits and circadian preference in Italian children and adolescents. "Sleep habits and circadian preference (morningness/ eveningness, M/E) have been extensively analyzed in adolescents and young adults, while few studies were conducted on children and early adolescents. Aim of the present study was to investigate the developmental changes of circadian preference and to analyze its relationship with sleep habits, sleep problems and circadian preference in a large sample by means of a school-based survey. One thousand seventy-three participants (50.8% boys and 49.2% girls; mean age = 10.6; range = 8-14 years), recruited from four schools randomly extracted within the district of Rome, completed a Standardized version of School Sleep Habits Survey developed by Carskadon et al. The questionnaire included items about sleep habits during schooldays and weekends; a Sleepiness Scale; a Sleep-Wake Problems Behaviour Scale; a Morningness/Eveningness scale. The results show a consistent age-related change in sleep habits, particularly in the weekends. The difference in sleep duration between schooldays and weekends increases linearly with age. No gender difference was observed in morningness/eveningness, while a significant linear increase in evening preference was found with increasing ages. M/E total scores correlated significantly with both self-reported sleep/wake problems and daytime sleepiness indicating a higher prevalence of sleep complaints in evening-type subjects. Overall, the present results support the existence of consistent age-related changes in sleep habits and M/E dimension in the 8- to 14-year age range". [92]

Luc ME, etal (2006) Characterization of symptoms of sleep disorders in children with headache. "To investigate the prevalence of sleep disorders and their symptoms in children with headaches, 64 patients in the outpatient clinics of the University Of Chicago Department Of Paediatric Neurology were interviewed. Investigated disorders included excessive daytime sleepiness, narcolepsy, insomnia, sleep apnoea, restlessness, and parasomnias. Unlike previous studies, subjects were compared with matched control patients by age and sex. Both headache and no headache groups completed a 111-item questionnaire detailing sleep symptoms and behaviours. It was found that children with headaches have a significantly higher prevalence of excessive daytime sleepiness, narcolepsy, and insomnia than children without headaches ($P < 0.005$), which is consistent with prior literature. A similar result was obtained in examining only migraines. However, we did not find a significantly higher prevalence of symptoms of sleep apnoea, restlessness, and parasomnias, which contradicts previous literature. Also, the effect of medications taken by headache patients as a confounding factor was insignificant. Overall, paediatricians may find it beneficial to ask about daytime sleepiness, narcolepsy, and insomnia when treating a headache patient". [93]

Heng K, Wirrell E. (2006) Sleep disturbance in children with migraine. "The objectives of this study were to determine if (1) children with migraine experience greater sleep disturbances than their siblings, (2) those with more severe migraine have greater levels of sleep disruption, and (3) these sleep disturbances lead to greater behavioural problems and more missed school. Children aged 6 to 18 years with a diagnosis of migraine for > 6 months, who had at least one sibling without migraine in the same age range, were identified through our neurology clinic database or at the time of the clinic visit. Parents completed the (1) demographic, general health, and migraine information questionnaire; (2) Child Sleep Habits Questionnaire; and (3) Behaviour Assessment System for Children: Second Edition (BASC-2) Parent Rating

Scales for each child. Cases with migraine had higher total sleep ($P < .02$), sleep delay ($P < .03$), and daytime sleepiness scores ($P < .001$) than controls. Cases with more severe migraines had higher total sleep ($P < .01$) and sleep duration scores ($P < .03$) than those with milder headaches. In cases, higher total sleep scores predicted greater behaviour problems on all four composite scales on the Behaviour Assessment System for Children: Second Edition (Externalizing Problems, $P < .05$; Internalizing Problems, $P < .005$; Behaviour Systems Index, $P < .003$; and Adaptability Skills, $P < .006$). We conclude that children with migraine are prone to greater sleep and behavioural disturbances than children without headache. Sleep disorders should be routinely queried and appropriate advice on sleep hygiene provided". [94]

Carotenuto M, etal (2005) Headache disorders as risk factors for sleep disturbances in school aged children. "Several epidemiological studies have shown the presence of co morbidity between various types of sleep disorders and different headache subtypes. Migraine without aura is a sensitive risk factor for disorders of initiating and maintaining sleep (odds ratio (OR) 8.2500), and chronic tension-type headache for sleep breathing disorders (OR 15.231), but headache disorder is a cumulative risk factor for disorders of excessive somnolence (OR 15.061). This result has not been reported in the clinical literature". [95]

Miller VA, etal(2003). "Migraine headaches and sleep disturbances in children. Parents reported a high rate of sleep disturbances in children, including sleeping too little (42%), bruxism (29%), child co-sleeping with parents (25%), and snoring (23%). Children with migraine headaches experienced more sleep disturbances compared to published healthy control norms. After controlling for child demographics, we found that the frequency and duration of migraine headaches predicted specific sleep disturbances, including sleep anxiety, parasomnias, and bedtime resistance. Children with migraine headaches have a high prevalence of sleep disturbances. The direction of the relationship between headaches and sleep is unknown. Regardless, interventions targeting sleep habits may improve headache symptoms, and effective treatment of headaches in children may positively impact sleep".[96]

Mohamad SS, etal (2021). Effect of Warm Water Foot Bath Therapy on Body Temperature among Children with Fever. Fever in children is a traditional warning for parents. The current study aimed to evaluate effect of warm water foot bath therapy on body temperature among children with fever. A quasi-experimental design was utilized. A purposeful sample of 100 children with fever in an outpatient clinic at Misr El-Hora general hospital participated in the current study. One tool used, child age, sex, diagnosis, use of antipyretics, use of antibiotics, baseline body temperature, and after application body temperature. The results revealed that near to three-quarters of the children in the study group return their body temperature to normal level versus more than one-third of the children in the control group after application with a statistically significant difference. The mean body temperature among children in the study group in the baseline was 38.7 ± .417 versus 38.6 ± .587 among children in the control group decreased to 37.4 ± .496 versus 37.8 ± .554 oC after application of warm water foot bath therapy respectively, with statistically significance difference. The current study concluded that applying warm water foot bath therapy in children with fever is effective in reducing body temperature than plain water compresses with statistically significant differences. Provide the hospital with written protocol on methods of warm water foot bath therapy to be applied in the hospitals was recommended [97]

"El-Naggar NS, Mohamed HR. (2020) Effectiveness of Warm Water Footbath on Temperature and Fatigue among Children with Fever. The mean score level of children's age was 10±1.3 & 10±1.5 years for both the study and control groups, respectively. Nearly two thirds of them (68% &62%) were boys in the study and control groups, respectively. There were significant differences in the temperature and fatigue score among children with a fever between the study and control groups after the application of warm water footbath therapy. Also, statistically significant differences between the children mean scores of temperature and fatigue pre- and post-footbath in the study group children. Warm water footbath is effective in reducing the temperature and fatigue level among children with fever. Recommendations: Warm water footbath should be involved in fever management protocol for children as a complementary therapy, and further studies with a large sample and another age group of children in another setting are also recommended". [98]

Another study revealed that there was a very high significant difference between the pre test and post test reduction in body temperature in the experimental group t value 8.068 at P value 0.0001. Also the significant difference of post test body temperature between the experimental and control group $t(58)=1.99$ at $p<0.05$ level of significance. The study showed that there was a significant association of pre-test body temperature of the experimental group with initial body temperature (($\chi 2=11.03$, $p<0.05$) and in control group with child's age and initial body temperature (($\chi 2=9.64$, 9.33, $p<0.05$). The result revealed that there is a significant association in post-test body temperature of the control group with child's age, gender and with initial body temperature (($\chi 2=10.93$, 3.59, 7.90 at $p<0.05$). Interpretation and Conclusion: The study concluded that there was a significant reduction in body temperature in the post test in the experimental group. This proved that the hot water foot bath therapy was effective in reduction of body temperature". [99]

Mandal I, Datta S, Ahmed N, De P. (2014) reported effectiveness of Warm Water Foot-Bath Therapy on Physiological Parameters of Children with Fever at a Selected Hospital, Kolkata, West Bengal. "Quasi-experimental study with non-equivalent control group time series design was conducted on warm water foot-bath therapy on 30 children with fever in the paediatric unit at Calcutta National Medical College and Hospital, Kolkata, by adopting non probability purposive sampling technique. The objectives of the study were to determine the effectiveness of warm water foot-bath therapy in terms of differences in physiological parameters of children with fever between experimental and control group. Physiological parameters were assessed before giving therapy, 15 and 25 min after therapy. Result showed an average reduction of physiological parameters, (i.e., axillary temperature, pulse rate, respiration rate, blood pressure) after giving warm water foot bath therapy in experimental group but in control group physiological parameters are significantly increased. Independent't' value among the mean physiological parameters between experimental and control group at 2nd observation, (i.e., 6.2, 2.13, 2.21, 0.39,

0.43 $p<0.05$) and at 3rd observation the computed't' values (16.5, 7.8, 5.84, 2.21, 2.15 $p<0.05$) were significant after warm water foot- bath therapy. The researcher recommended further studies with large sample, also with other age group of children, wide range of axillary temperature, more number of observations, comparative study between warm water foot bath therapy and other types of hydrotherapy, comparative study between warm water foot bath therapy and use of antipyretics, effect of warm water foot bath therapy on other physiological parameter like oxygen saturation etc".[100]

RESEARCH GAP ANALYSIS

Sleep allows the body to preserve energy, restore normal functions, support physical growth, and enhance mental development. The most well-known symptom of insufficient sleep is daytime tiredness. Sleepiness in youngsters, on the other hand, often emerges as irritability, behavioural issues, learning challenges, adolescent car accidents, and low academic performance. [6–8]

Sleep difficulties are widespread in children and adolescence, and they're linked to neuro cognitive and psychosocial problems, as well as increased caregiver stress. Sleep disorders may manifest themselves in a variety of ways in babies, children, and teenagers, frequently resulting in major deficits in several domains of daily functioning. While bedtime settling problems and frequent overnight awakenings are more common in infancy and early childhood, sleep problems caused by poor sleep hygiene or circadian rhythm disturbances are more frequent in adolescents. In children and teenagers, the onset of particular sleep disorders may exacerbate any underlying co-morbid medical conditions like obesity and asthma, as well as psychological issues like sadness, anxiety, and drug misuse. According to current data, persistently interrupted sleep in children and teenagers may cause cognitive difficulties such as attention, learning, and memory. Behavioural therapies for paediatric sleep difficulties (e.g., progressive extinction, parent education, good bedtime rituals) have been demonstrated to improve clinically relevant outcomes, particularly in young children. This is especially important considering the scarcity of evidence on the use of pharmaceutical therapies in children with sleep problems.

As the circadian rhythm is established, the number of night-time awakenings gradually decreases over the first year of life. Therefore, whereas a 1-month-old infant wakens 2 or 3 times per night, a 12-month-old infant usually does not wake up more than 2 times per night.[6] However, brief awakenings that follow the sleep cycle (90–120 min) continue to occur, with the child normally falling back to sleep without external intervention.[7]

Sleep disorders are prevalent in the paediatric age range.[8] It is estimated that until adolescence, 20%–30% of children present some sleep abnormality, and this prevalence is higher among children with neuropsychiatric comorbidities.[9] On the other hand, sleep disorders may also in themselves increase the risk that a series of metabolic and behavioural changes may emerge, leading to attention deficits, mood disorders, weight gain, and even neuro-developmental alterations.[10, 11]

Because sleep is such a complicated process, there are several elements that might influence its quality. Fig. 1 represents the factor potentially influencing sleep in the hospital setting.

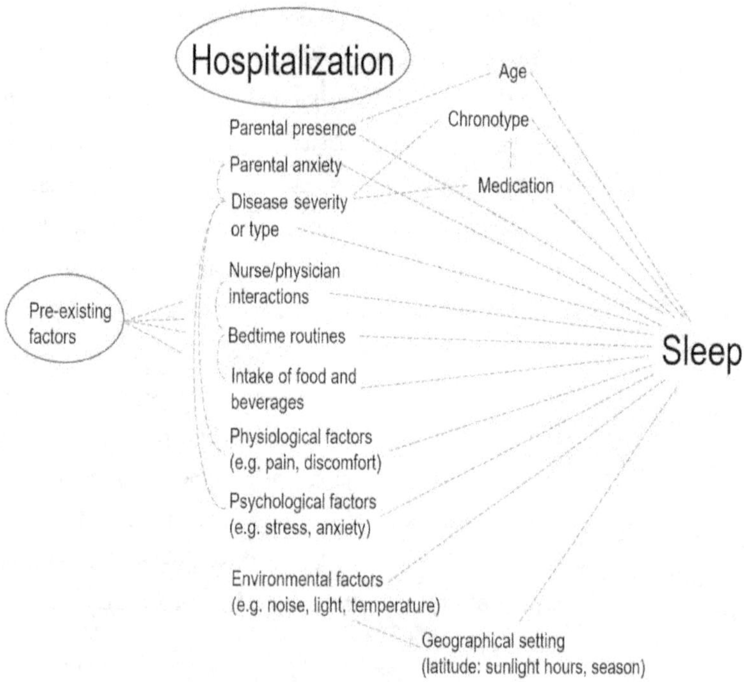

Figure 2. Factors potentially influencing sleep in a hospital setting

Over-sedation, hallucination, ataxia, short-term memory impairment, disorientation, respiratory depression, and depression are all side effects of using these medicines often.

There have been research that suggest the BEARS sleep problem questionnaire is reliable and valid in children and adolescents from Bogotá, Colombia. Sleep is critical for school-aged children's health and well-being. The purpose of this study was to examine the BEARS questionnaire's reliability and content validity in children and adolescents aged 9 to 17. In Bogotá, Colombia, the poll included 8,862 children and adolescents from 24 recognised educational institutions. Participants were given the BEARS questionnaire in a structured, self-administered format. "A sub-sample of 246 people was used to conduct reliability tests. The consistency, construct validity, and reliability of the instrument were assessed using Cronbach's alpha coefficient, exploratory factor analysis (EFA), and the weighted Kappa coefficient. The findings showed acceptable consistency and reliability (global Cronbach's alpha = 0.732; range = 0.706 to 0.769). (Kappa = 0.665; range = 0.706–0.769) The EFA found a single factor (item 1: sleep troubles) that explained 61.4 percent of the variance by combining two interactions 2/gl = 2690.817; p = 0.001. The BEARS questionnaire's internal consistency, reliability, and validity were all good. As a result of these results, this instrument is largely recommended for use in primary care in Bogotá, Colombia, for investigating and screening sleep disorders in school-aged populations". 59

The following gap was identified in the available literature:

There are no studies found regarding the different therapies for the children having early sleep onset problem. So there is an importance to provide non-pharmacological and non-invasive intervention to provide good sleep during hospitalization.

Because it soothes the body and mind, a hot water foot bath promotes restful sleep. It works by slightly boosting the body temperature before gradually lowering it after 15 minutes. Indirectly, this might help you sleep. The gradual decline in body temperature makes us tired, and we feel better prepared for sleep as a result. A heated footbath also redirects blood from the head to the lower body, lowering brain activity and simulating the pre-sleep state.

A warm-water footbath is a wet heat application that is applied locally. It is a simple and non-invasive treatment that may be used at home. It might be a non-pharmaceutical technique of assisting patients with exhaustion and sleep issues while in the hospital.

Sleep disruption is said to be a major issue for children in hospitals. Despite the fact that sleep drugs have a lot of adverse effects, footbath has been discovered to be a potent alternative therapy for sleep induction.

According to a new study, poor sleep patterns are highly prevalent among hospitalised patients, and this can contribute to a variety of health issues. Warm water foot baths are believed to be one of the most efficient ways for inducing sleep among hospitalised patients. A heated footbath increases vascular dilatation and heat dissipation by warming the epidermis. The subject's sleeping pattern will be improved by an intervention that improves heat dissipation prior to sleep.

Although, there are numerous therapeutic options available for improving quality of sleep among hospitalized patients. An effective mean with the least adverse effect is required in children due to a reduced immunization shield. As per our knowledge in the available literature, data of effectiveness of warm foot bath on quality of sleep among hospitalized patients is scarce. Additionally, there were no such studies available among hospitalized children. Hence, researcher decided to evaluate the effectiveness of warm foot bath in promotion of early sleep onset among hospitalized children.

	Author	Research focus	Conclusion by author
disturbance & gical distress hospitalized in India sleep ice in zation in india	Ramya samarth 2021	Parental perception on pediatric inpatient experienced that their children get disturbances overnight in the hospital.	Child centered intervention may improve sleep & dec psychological distress among children.

Article	Author	Research focus	Conclusion by author	Remarks of the scholar
Behavioral intervention for sleep problems in childhood a Brazilian randomized controlled trial Behavioural inteervention.pdf	Mindell & Moore, 2014	Sixty-two children with bedtime problems and night waking in hospital were randomized to a parent-based intervention	Behavioral parent-based intervention is effective in improving the quality of sleep and the diurnal behavior of children.	The study was effective improving sleep quality and daytime behavior of children. The present study intervention different

- Incidence of sleep disturbances in children during hospitalization is 52.3% in India.
- Studies reported the sleep quality but no intervention has been administered.
- Some studies show that behavioral educational intervention for sleep problems in childhood & parent based intervention were given but child centered intervention will improve child's sleep more than parent education.
- There is record of other therapies & interventions for children with sleep disturbances but no study is found in India related to warm foot bath in hospitalized children.
- Studies showed effectiveness of warm foot bath in various conditions as fever, anxiety, psychological distress but no study related to sleep in hospitalized children.

- Hence, researcher decided to evaluate the effectiveness of warm foot bath in promotion of early sleep onset among hospitalized children which is non-pharmacological, non invasive, cost effective intervention for children.

Research Question

Whether the warm foot bath is efficacious in promotion of early sleep onset among hospitalized children?

Anticipated Translatory Component

1. Innovation of administration of warm foot bath in promotion of early sleep onset among hospitalized children.
2. Warm foot bath can be included as a standard operating procedure for the children in hospital care.
3. Warm foot bath helps to promote health.
4. It will enhance knowledge of community regarding well defined warm bath procedure.

PICOT FORMAT

Population- Children of age group 4yr to 12 yrs

Intervention- Warm foot bath

Control Group- Hospital standard care

Outcome- Promotion of early sleep onset

Conceptual Framework

It's a framework that instructs the investigator on how to proceed with the study's objectives based on the model. It is a scientific portrayal of the study's phases, activities, and results. A conceptual frame work is made up of a set of concepts and prepositions that define their connection. The main goal is to generalise and make scientific results relevant. The theory's building pieces are concepts.

"Conceptualization is a process of forming ideas which utilizes and forms a conceptual frame work for the study. It is the abstract, logical structure which enables the researcher to link the findings to the nursing body of knowledge. A framework is the abstract of logical structure of meaning that guides the development of the study and the body of knowledge. Conceptual framework of this study was based on the helping art in clinical nursing theory by Ernestine Wieden Bach in 1964. The theory focuses on three concepts such as identification, ministration and validation".

In Identification Demographic data of the child is collected as: Age of the child, Gender, Educational background, Duration of sleep, Day of hospitalization, Dietary pattern, Previous history of hospitalization, Type of disease, Nature of disease., Standardized Bears scale for the assessment of early sleep onset, Structured observational checklist for the observation of the early sleep onset of the child .

In ministration warm foot bath is administered to the experimental group for 3 subsequent days 20 min before 20 min of sleep and routine care to the control group.

In validation Assessment of early sleep onset on first and final day in experimental and control group by using Standardized BEARS SCALE and structured observational checklist for the improvement in early sleep onset in hospitalized children.

FIGURE 3: ERNESTINE WIEDENBACH'S THEORY IN1964 CONCEPTUAL FRAMWEORK

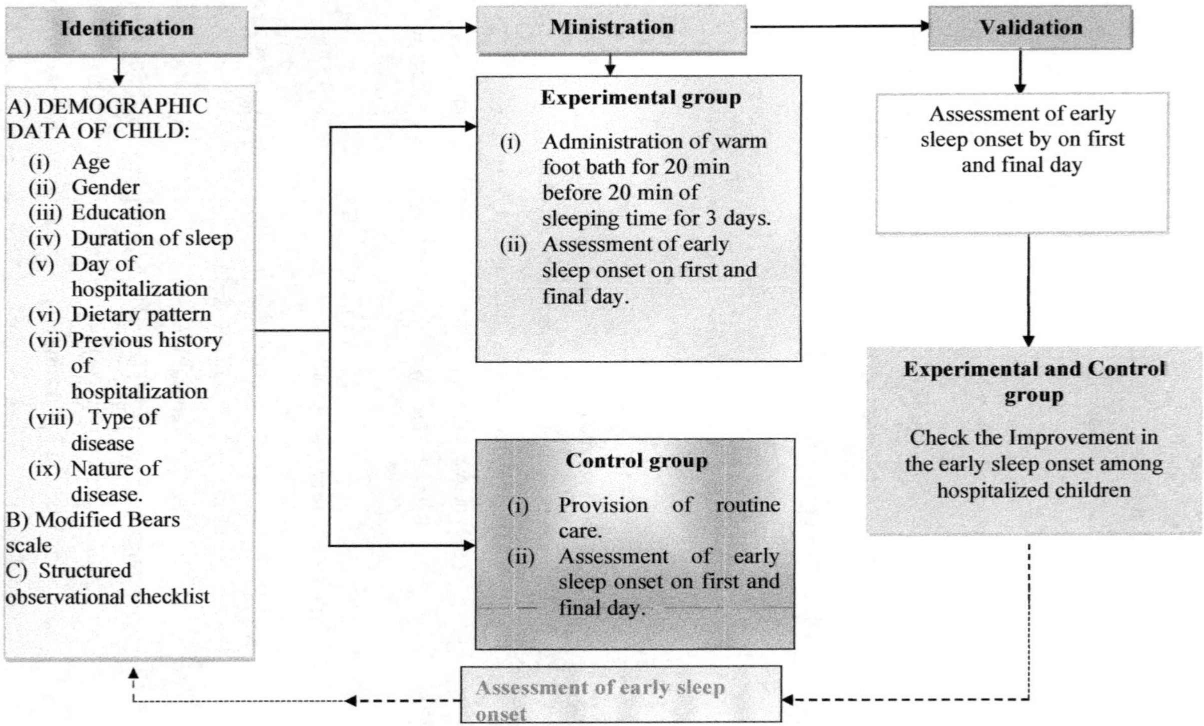

RESEARCH DESIGN

Research Approach: Interventional Evaluatory Approach.

A research design serves the purpose to create an evidence to get answers to the research questions in an effective manner.

Research designs provide the blue print for the study. The researcher decides this blue print based on what is the type of inquiry in the research.

In this study researcher used Randomized Controlled Trial Research design

Aim

The aim of the study is to evaluate the efficacy of warm foot bath in promotion of early sleep onset among hospitalized children.

Objectives of the study

1. To assess the existing pattern of early sleep onset of the experimental and control group.
2. To assess the efficacy of warm foot bath on promotion of early sleep onset at experimental group.
3. To evaluate the efficacy of warm foot bath on promotion of early sleep onset between the experimental and control group.
4. To compare the efficacy of warm foot bath on promotion of early sleep onset between the experimental and control group.
5. To associate the warm foot bath with their selected demographic variables.

Type and Nature of the study

The study is interventional analytical in which researcher is administering the warm foot bath to hospitalized children who are fulfilling inclusion and exclusion stated criteria and the effect on early sleep onset is tested. This intervention WARM FOOT BATH is non-invasive and non-pharmaceutical effect which is best in economically needs very less budget, there is no adverse and side effect for this. This can be given by caretaker needs very small information no need of training. This can be used at home setting. This will help to use this intervention as an integral part in promotion of early onset of sleep in the practices in hospitalized child care. It can be included in evidence-based Practice. This study results can be used to make new protocol and policies related to child care. This may the cost-effective intervention to improve sleep pattern in hospitalized child health. The public may be made aware regarding effectiveness of warm foot bath related to sleep. The study may generate the future hypothesis to conduct the longitudinal research study.

The community nurse may get opportunity to arrange mass education awareness program regarding effectiveness of warm foot bath.

Nature of the study

The researcher adopted the Randomised control trail- time series research design for the current research. In this the researcher utilized the simple random sampling technique for the sample selection. Researcher had utilized the following stapes for the collection of data: The investigator approached the Children admitted in the hospital. Took the informed consent form the children and their parents. The socio demographic data was collected by interviewing the patients and was noted in the proforma. Assess the early sleep onset in both the groups. Application of warm foot bath therapy to the children in the experimental group and assess the early sleep onset on first day and final day of data collection. Compared the effectiveness of both in intervention. The association of outcome of early sleep onset with selected demographic variables in both the groups.

This study has a great scope as follows:

The study result will help to use this intervention as an integral part in promotion of early onset of sleep in the practices in hospitalized child care.

It can be included in evidence-based Practice.

It can minimize the risk for ill health among children related to sleep disturbance.

This study results can be used to make new protocol and policies related to child care.

This study can be clinically recommended as diagnosing children for ill-health.

This may the cost-effective intervention to improve sleep pattern in hospitalized child health.

The public may be made aware regarding effectiveness of warm foot bath related to sleep.

The study may generate the future hypothesis to conduct the longitudinal research study.

The study may generate the future hypothesis to conduct the research study for all groups of children.

The community nurse may get opportunity to arrange mass education awareness program regarding effectiveness of warm foot bath.

GROUP	**PRE TEST**	**INTERVENTION & OBSEVATION**					**POST TES**
		First day		Second day		Third day	
Experimental group	OB	X1	O1	X2	02	X2	O3
Control group	OB	Hospital standardized care	O1	Hospital standardized care	O2	Hospital standardized care	O3

KEY

OB: pre test with STANDARDIZED BEARS SCALE & STRUCTURED OBSEVATIONAL CHECK LIST

XI, X2, X3: ADMINISTRATION OF WARM FOOT BATH TO EXPERIMENTAL GROUP for Consecutive 3 Days

O1, O2, O3: Post test after each intervention with same STANDARDIZED BEARS SCALE & STRUCTURED OBSEVATIONAL CHECK LIST.

Hospital standardized care: for control group

Commensurate Sample Size

The sample size calculation is very important in the whole planning of the study. It should be representative to extrapolate the findings of the outcome of the study being undertaken. The sample size for the study was calculated using following formula to obtain a sample size that is best representative of the population.

Using following formula to obtain a sample size that is best representative of the population.

Formula:

Formula

$$n \geq \frac{Z^2_{1-\frac{\alpha}{2}} \times P \times (1-p)}{d^2}$$

α :Type I error at 5 % l.o.s. = 1.96

β: Type II Error at 20% (1-β) = 0.8

Estimated Proportion (p) = (Ref article)

Estimation of Error d = 10%

$N = 1.96 * 0.76*(0.24)/(0.10)^2 = 71$

Formula

Sample size Formula For Superiority trial (one-tail)

$$n \geq \frac{Z^2_{1-\frac{\alpha}{2}} \times \sigma^2}{d^2}$$

α :Type I error at 5 % l.o.s. = 1.96

β: Type II Error at 20% (1-β) = 0.8

Estimated Standard Deviation (σ) = (11/200)*100=0.59 (Ref article)

Estimation of Error d = 10%

$N = ((1.96)^2 \times 0.05) / (0.05)^2$

=

Sample size Formula For Superiority trial (one-tail)

$$n_1 = n_2 = \frac{2(z_\alpha + z_\beta)^2\sigma^2}{(\epsilon - \delta)^2} =$$

$Z\alpha$: Type I error for superiority one tail at 5% = 1.64

Z_β :Type II error for superiority one tail at 5% = 1.28

ε : - True Mean Difference at before and after value =(0.44) from reference article with std.dev. = 0.98.(Reference article : Effect of footbath on sleep quality of elderly :A blinded randomized clinical trial

δ = 0.1

Clinically relevant (ε-δ) : = (-0.44 –(-1)) = (-0.45) Reducing the scale .

(N) = (2 x(1.64 +1.28)*0.98)/0.45^2 = 58.2 ≅ 60 in each group

Variables

The variables included in the research are:

Confound Variable

1) When the mother is with child.

2) When child is suffering with chronic illnesses.

3) Protein energy malnutrition.

4) Child is experiencing any kind of physical pain.

SCHEMETIC DIGRAM OF REASERCH DESIGN

STUDY APPROACH
Interventional Evaluatory Approach

STUDY DESIGN
Randomized Controlled Trial

PARTICIPANTS
Children fulfils inclusion criteria admitted in hospital.

SAMPLING TECHNIQUES
Probability: Simple Random sampling computer generated method

SAMPLE SIZE
120 patients (60 FOR GROUP I & 60 FOR GROUP II)

DATA COLLECTION TOOL
Standardized BEARS scale for assessment of sleep, structured Observational checklist, warm foot bath

VARIABLES

CONFOUND VERIABLES

DATA COLLECTION

Analysis-Descriptive and inferential statistics

DATA COLLECTION

PHASE	ACTIVITY	DAY	DETAILS
Phase 1 PLANNING PHASE	Selection of sample	DAY 1-	Introduction to parent/ caretaker regarding procedure. Ensure willingness consent for involvement in study
			Randomization : computer generated simple randomization for experimental and control group
	Collection of Demographic Data	DAY1	Collection of Data with the help of structured demographic questionnaire
	PRETEST	DAY1	Data collection with the help of Standardized BEARS Scale , Structured observational check list
Intervention	WARM FOOT BATH	DAY1	Administration of warm foot bath for the duration of 20 min before the 20 min of sleep time . No intervention for control group – standard hospital care
		DAY 2	Administration of warm foot bath for the duration of 20 min before the 20 min of sleep time . No intervention for control group – standard hospital care
		DAY 3	Administration of warm foot bath for

			the duration of 20 min before the 20 min of sleep time . No intervention for control group – standard hospital care
EVALUATION PHASE	POST TEST	10 min	Data collection with the help of Standardized BEARS Scale , Structured observational check list

METHODOLOGY

Research Setting: The setting of the study was pediatric wards of the VINOBA BHAVE RURAL HOSPITL SAWANGI MEGHE.

Study Design: A research design serves the purpose to create evidence to get answers to the research questions in an effective manner. Research designs provide the blueprint for the study. The researcher decides this blueprint based on what is the type of inquiry in the research. This was a Randomized controlled trial study.

Figure 4: Randomized controlled trial

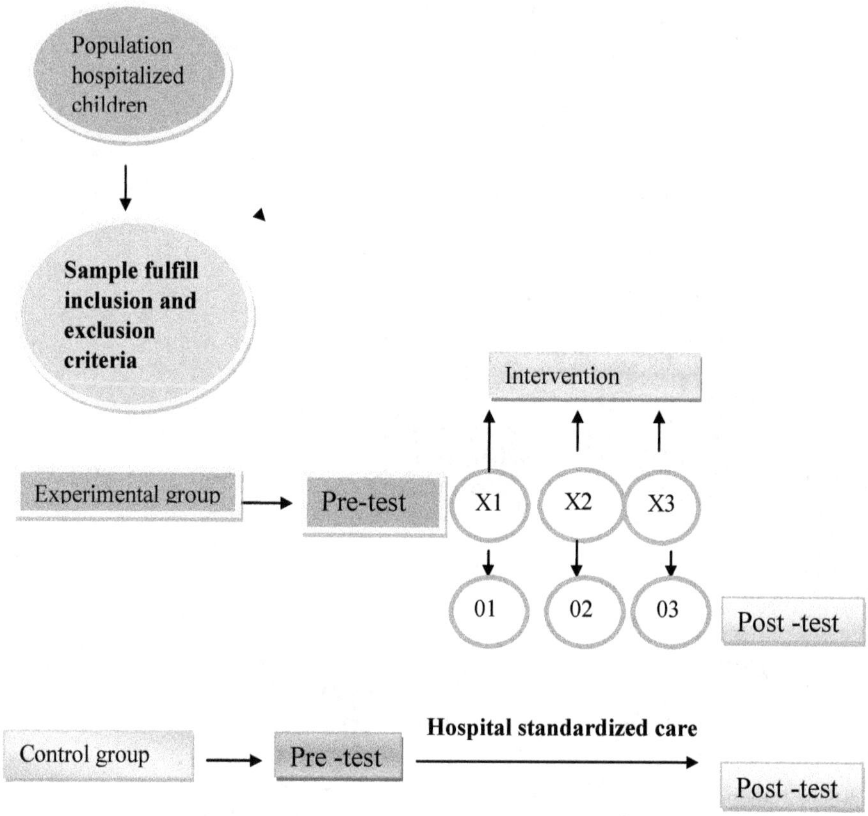

CONSORT 2010 Flow Diagram

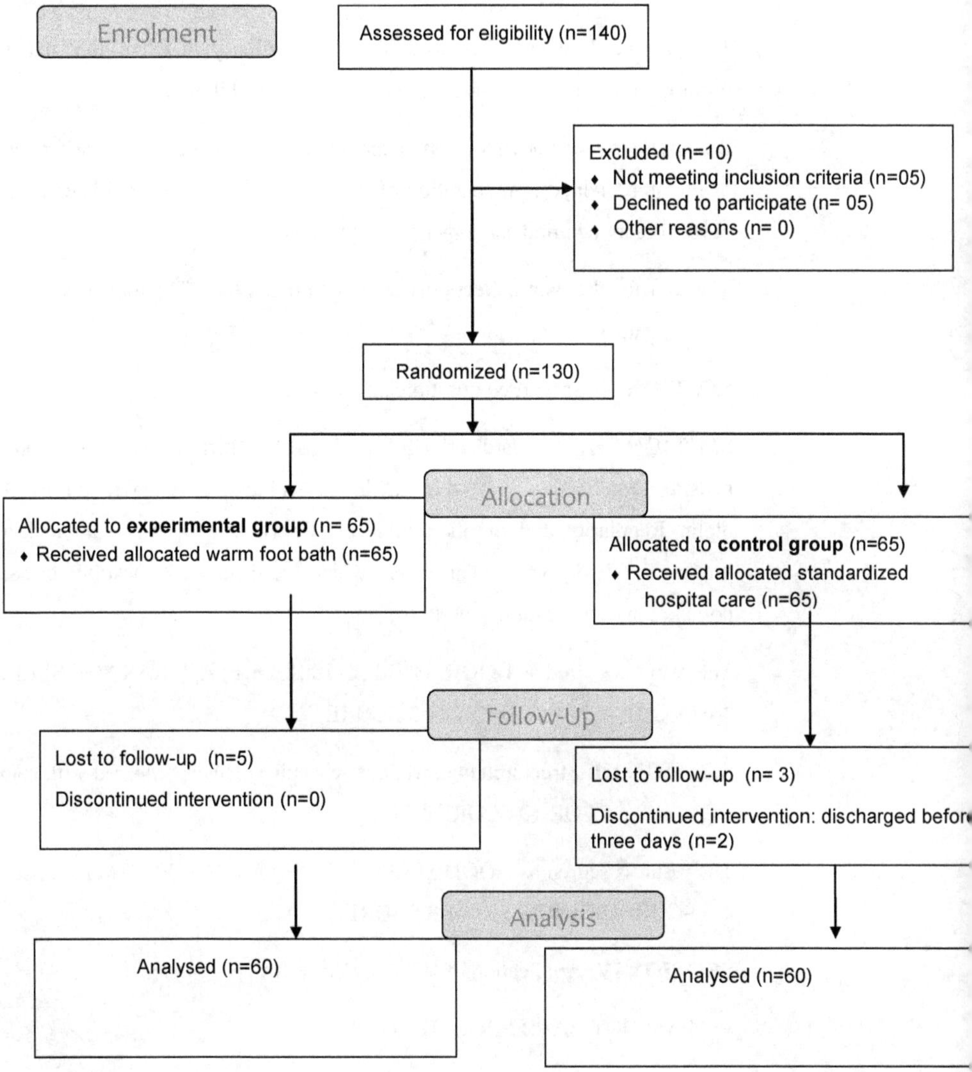

Participants: The participants of the research were the children admitted to the pediatric ward of the selected hospital of the selected city.

Sampling Techniques: The sampling techniques used in the study were the probability: Computer generated Random Sampling technique.

Material with their standardization:

The present study is aimed to evaluate the efficacy of warm foot bath in promotion of early sleep onset among hospitalized children.

Researcher's own knowledge and experience, expert's suggestions and review of literature helped in preparation of the tool. Tool was prepared keeping the objectives in the mind and expert's suggestions.

The tool for the data collection was Standardized tool. The tool used in this study includes:

SECTION –I: Structured questionnaire

SECTION- II: Standardized BEARS SCALE which includes 5 domains bedside problems. Excessive daytime sleepiness, Awakening during the night, Regularity and duration of sleep, Snoring. Tool was validated for scoring in this 5 domains considered which are included 2 questions in each domain total 10 questions; marks10.

The result is scored as GOOD SLEEP: 7-10 SCORE, AVERARAGE SLEEP: 4-6 SCORE & POOR SLEEP: 1-3 SCORE.

SECTION III: Structured observational checklist. This is prepared with some 10 parameters FOR 10 SCORE

The result is scored as GOOD SLEEP; 7-10 SCORE, AVERARAGE SLEEP: 4-6 SCORE, POOR SLEEP: 1-3 SCORE.

SECTION IV: Application of WARM FOOT BATH

WARM FOOT BATH PROCEDURE

Preliminary assessment of child

1. Assess the child for preparedness of sleep
2. Assess the general condition of child

3. Prepare mother for the procedure so she can cooperate for the procedure and give her time upto complete of procedure.

Preparation of the Equipment for procedure

1. Five-litre foot bucket
2. Bath Thermometer to test that the water is between 100° and 115° F (43°C- 46°C)
3. Sheet or blanket
4. Dry bath towel
5. Material for protection of the bed, if needed
6. Pitcher or mug to add hot water.

Important Considerations

1. Do not use hot foot bath on patients with diabetes or peripheral vascular disease unless the temperature is low; maximum 103°F (39°C) Be careful to not burn the patient when adding hot water
2. Use cold compress to head when oral temperature exceeds 100° F (38°C), or when patient begins sweating

Treatment:

1) Explain procedure to the patient
2)Have room warm and free of drafts
3) Assemble the materials
4)Protect the bedding, if needed
5)Drape the blankets over a chair or spread on a bed
6) Fill bucket with water 100° F to 115° F (43°C- 46°C) high enough to cover ankles and check temperature of water with bath thermometer
7) Assist patient in undressing and wrap in sheet
8) Wrap dry bath towel around patient's neck to catch sweat and prevent escape of body heat
9) Assist patient to place feet in bucket. Reassure patient by putting your hands in the water first

10) Wrap the dry bath towel one at a time around the patient, enclosing the bucket to allow heat to build up

11) Add hot water as patient can tolerate it, up to 120° F (49°C

12) Continue treatment for 20 minutes before 20 min of sleeping time.

13) Raise feet out of tub, dry feet, legs and thighs, dress in bed clothes

14 Put thick, warm socks on the patient, allowing them to rest in bed.

After care of article:

1. Dispose water in a utility area.
2. Wash bucket with disinfectant solution
3. Ask mother to give comfortable position to child
4. Observe the child for sleep onset

http://amazinghealth.com/AH-health-hot-bath-blood-feet

PILOT STUDY

Pilot Study was conducted on 10% of the main study sample from the selected areas. The pilot study period was from **10/12/2019 to 15/12/2019.**

Validity and Reliability of Tools: Tools were submitted to ten experts in the field of child health nursing, Community health nursing, Medical-Surgical Nursing, and Statistics to test the content validity. Modifications were carried out according to the recommendations of experts on clarity of tools and appropriateness and completeness of the content". By using PEARSON'S TEST-RETEST METHOD the reliability of the tool was found reliable with hence the tools were found valid and reliable.

		Mean	Standard deviation	Standard error mean	95% Confidence Interval of the Difference	DF	Significant 2 tailed
Pair 1	OBSERVATIONAL CHECKLIST POST TEST - OBSERVATIONAL CHECKLIST PRE TEST	2.100	1.729	.547	.863	3.337	3.841
Pair 2	Structured BEARS SCALE post test & pre test	.900	.738	.233	.372	1.428	3.857

There is a significant mean difference between experimental pre test observational and post test observational as the calculated T value of 3.841 is more than the T table value of 2.26 at 0.05 level of significance. Similarly there is a significant mean difference between experimental pre test bears scale and post test bears scale as the calculated T value of 3.857 is more than the T table value of 2.26 at 0.05 level of significance

Methods with justification

The children were selected with computer generated random sampling methods. The participants willing to participate in this study were explained about the study and their role in it. Their doubts were clarified and informed written consent was taken from them.. The data was collected from the samples.

DATA COLLECTION PROCESS:

The research study proposal was presented and approved by

Institutional Ethical Committee, DMIMS (DU)/IEC/2018-19/715902/04/2018 and Doctoral Research Committee, DMIMS/ Ph.D.Regn/2018/248 Date 24/04/2018 of Datta Meghe Institute of Medical Sciences (Deemed to be university) Wardha.

DATA collection process is divided into three phases

PLANNING PHASE

The permission was obtained from chief medical superintendent of Acharya Vinoba Bhave Rural hospital Sawangi (Meghe) Dist Wardha with letter ref no: SRMMCON/ 21-22/117 DATED 23/07/2021 before proceeding to data collection process. Data collection process carried out from period **27.08.2021 to 13.12.2021.**

Samples are selected for both experimental & control group by computer generated randomization that fulfils the inclusion criteria

Researcher obtained informed written consent of the sample's parent with the help of a consent form for every sample of both group.

IMPLEMENTATION PHASE

- The demographic data collected with the structured validated questionnaire.
- Assessment of existing pattern of early sleep onset of experimental & control group with the help of Standardized BEARS SCALE & structured observational check list.

- Administration of warm foot bath for 20 min before 20 min going to bed for 3 days continuously for experimental group.

EVALUATION PHASE

- Assess the onset of sleep with the help of Standardized BEARS scale & structured observational checklist in control group samples for the first day considered as existing pattern of the children early sleep onset
- Assessment the effect of warm foot bath on the promotion of onset of sleep with the help of a structured observational checklist & Standardized BEARS scale every day after intervention.
- Compare the result of warm foot bath on the promotion of early onset of sleep in the experimental group.
- Compare the result of post test on the promotion of sleep in experimental & control group.
- Find out the association between warm foot baths with the selected demographic variables of samples in both groups.

Ethical considerations

1. Approval obtained from ethical committee before commencement of study.
2. Permission from the competent authority was obtained before the study.
3. Informed consent of the sample taken prior to the study.
4. Confidentiality of data and the privacy of the sample maintained.
5. Participants were given full rights to ask questions about any additional information.
6. Participants were given freedom to leave from the study at any stage without giving any reason to the investigator.
7. Self-respect and dignity of the samples maintained during the study.

Plan for data analysis

- The collected data was analyzed using descriptive and inferential statistics like frequency, percentage, mean, SD, chi-squire, t test. The analyzed data was presented in the form of tables, and figures.

Eligibility criteria

Inclusion Criteria includes

- The children admitted in hospital
- Children age group 4 year to 12 years
- Who are willing to participate in the study
- Who understands the instructions given in Marathi English or Hindi

Exclusion criteria included

- Children on intravenous infusion on lower limb.
- Children suffering with cardio vascular diseases.
- Children who are on sedatives.
- The children suffering with convulsive disorder.
- The unconscious children.
- Who is mentally challenged
- Parents are not willing for treatment
- Having paralyzed extremities
- Child having diabetes

ANALYSIS OF RESULT & DISSCUSSION

Data Analysis in tabular form

Statistical analysis helps scientists are able to make excellent sense of quantitative info. Without data, quantitative details shall be regarded as a chaotic mass of figures. A descriptive index originating from a test is recognized as being a statistic.

Examination will be the procedure of planning and synthesizing the information to answer research questions and also test hypothesis, as well that is a method of systematically applying statistical methods to describe, summarize and also compare information. In the present study, quantitative analysis technique is used. Quantitative analysis is a highly systematic and organized process. It deals with analyzing numerical values using statistical techniques for describing and explaining the research outcome. In other words, quantitative analysis uses numerical data to describe and interpret the results. Because numerically interpreted data are provided for quantitative analysis, data collection efficiency, data entry precision and the suitability of an analytical method play an important role in drawing reliable conclusions.

The evaluation of research data offers the outcomes of the research. These results have been analyzed and interpreted, providing problem to the aims of the job, the theoretical time frame of its, today's body of comparable research knowledge, as well as boundaries of the adopted exploration strategies, of theirs, (two) their significance, (three) the importance of theirs, (four) the degree to which they could be generalized, as well as (five) the implications of theirs.

Trustworthiness of the outcomes among the initial interpretive jobs is analyzing whether the outcomes are correct. This evaluation, in turn, involves an extensive evaluation of the study's conceptual limitations as well as methodologic. In taking a look at the believability of results, researchers seek to create various kinds of evidence. One form of proof is from last exploration on the subject. Investigators should take a look at whether their results are in line with those of various other studies; if you're about to find discrepancies, an extensive evaluation of the options for any variations need to be undertaken. Evidence could typically be created through peripheral specifics analyses, several of which are talked about earlier in this chapter. For instance, scientists are able to have much better confidence within the accuracy of the findings providing they've realized that their procedures are dependable as well as have ruled at bay biases. It's really useful to do a strength analysis when the outcomes of statistical tests aren't statistically significant.

The area of results for an investigation will be the knowledge section of the report which will be where the descriptive and inferential mathematical tests show their objective evidence and/or statistics. The data contribute to creating new information and facts and to avoid knowledge stagnation.

Analysis is the method of arranging data synthetization in order to address research questions and test the hypothesis. The study aims to minimize the data in an accessible way so that testing problem collection can be examined and evaluated.

Analysis and interpretation studies that comprise the grouping, labelling, and tabulation of details required to conduct quantitative or qualitative analyzes as per the scope of the sample and necessary for the results. Analysis of the data follows information collection and follows its interpretation or application.

Analysis is described as "the categorizing, organizing, manipulation and summarizing of the data in order to reduce it to an intelligible and interpretable form, so that the research problem can be studied and tested, including the relation between the variables."

DATA ANALYSIS AND INTERPRETATION

Introduction

Statistical analysis helps scientists are able to make excellent sense of quantitative info. Without data, quantitative details shall be regarded as a chaotic mass of figures. A descriptive index originating from a test is recognized as being a statistic.

Examination will be the procedure of planning and synthesizing the information to answer research questions and also test hypothesis, as well that is a method of systematically applying statistical methods to describe, summarize and also compare information. In the present study, quantitative analysis technique is used. Quantitative analysis is a highly systematic and organized process. It deals with analyzing numerical values using statistical techniques for describing and explaining the research outcome. In other words, quantitative analysis uses numerical data to describe and interpret the results. Because numerically interpreted data are provided for quantitative analysis, data collection efficiency, data entry precision and the suitability of an analytical method play an important role in drawing reliable conclusions.

The evaluation of research data offers the outcomes of the research. These results have been analyzed and interpreted, providing problem to the aims of the job, the theoretical time frame of its, today's body of comparable research knowledge, as well as boundaries of the adopted exploration strategies, of theirs, (two) their significance, (three) the importance of theory (four) the degree to which they could be generalized, as well as (five) the implications of theirs.

Trustworthiness of the outcomes among the initial interpretive jobs is analyzing whether the outcomes are correct. This evaluation, in turn, involves an extensive evaluation of the study's conceptual limitations as well as methodological. In taking a look at the believability of results, researchers seek to create various kinds of evidence. One form of proof is from last exploration on the subject. Investigators should take a look at whether their results are in line with those of various other studies; if you're about to find discrepancies, an extensive evaluation of the options for any variations need to be undertaken. Evidence could typically be created through peripheral specifics analyses, several of which are talked about earlier in this chapter. For instance, scientists are able to have much better confidence within the accuracy of the findings providing they've realized that their procedures are dependable as well as have ruled at bay biases. It's really useful to do a strength analysis when the outcomes of statistical tests aren't statistically significant.

The area of results for an investigation will be the knowledge section of the report which will be where the descriptive and inferential mathematical tests show their objective evidence and/or statistics. The data contribute to creating new information and facts and to avoid knowledge stagnation.

Analysis is the method of arranging data synthetization in order to address research questions and test the hypothesis. The study aims to minimize the data in an accessible way so that testing problem collection can be examined and evaluated.

Analysis and interpretation studies that comprise the grouping, labelling, and tabulation of details required to conduct quantitative or qualitative analyzes as per the scope of the sample and necessary for the results. Analysis of the data follows information collection and follows its interpretation or application.

Analysis is described as "the categorizing, organizing, manipulation and summarizing of the data in order to reduce it to an intelligible and interpretable form, so that the research problem can be studied and tested, including the relation between the variables."

In the present study data collected for main study was for the period **23/07/2021,** research scholar collected data related to objectives of the study which are well defined. Include total120 participants from ACHARYA VINOBA BHAVE RURAL HOSPITAL SAWANG the sample is divided into 2 group control group (60) and experimental group (60). Details of demographic and other characteristics are given below.

CRITICAL APPRAISAL OF THE STUDY

Extent of Research Gap filled

Sleep difficulties are widespread in children and adolescence, and they're linked to neuro- cognitive and psychosocial problems, as well as increased caregiver stress. Sleep disorders may manifest themselves in a variety of ways in babies, children, and teenagers, frequently resulting in major deficits in several domains of daily functioning. While bedtime settling problems and frequent overnight awakenings are more common in infancy and early childhood, sleep problems caused by poor sleep hygiene or circadian rhythm disturbances are more common in adolescents.

The onset of particular sleep disorders in children and teenagers may exacerbate any underlying medical disease, such as obesity or asthma, as well as psychological issues, such as sadness, anxiety, and drug misuse. Chronically interrupted sleep in children and teenagers has been linked to issues with attention, learning, and memory, according to current research. Behavioral therapies for pediatric sleep difficulties (e.g., graded extinction, parent education, good bedtime rituals) have been demonstrated to result in clinically significant improvements, particularly in young children. This is especially critical considering the scarcity of evidence on the use of pharmaceutical therapies in children with sleep problems.

Sleep is important for a child's growth and development, and sleep patterns may be seen in foetuses as early as 26 weeks. 1 Sleep characteristics vary dramatically throughout the first year of life, and then develop over the length of childhood. 2Newborns have an ultradian sleep pattern, with frequent awakenings due to hunger and pain rather than the time of day, but 1-year-old babies have a well-established circadian cycle.[3]

Sleep duration over 24 hours in newborns ranges from 14 to 17 hours, declines to 11–14 hours during the first and second years of life, and then drops to 10–13, 9–11, and 8–10 hours in pre-schoolers, school-aged children, and teenagers, respectively. 4 The decrease in total sleep happens mostly owing to shorter daytime sleep hours throughout the early years of life. In this manner, a 1-month-old newborn's sleep is dispersed around half of the time throughout the day, but a 12-month-old infant would have 1 or 2 1.5-hour daytime sleep periods. By the age of five, the need for daytime sleep has vanished, with the morning nap being the first to go.[5]

Limitations of the present study

No one was blinded.

Selection of sample as per the day of hospitalization.

Bias limitation.

If mother is with child then child sleeps well

Immediate post-doctoral research direction & Suggested future studies

1. Large scale study can be done.
2. Community based study can be done
3. RCT with another traditional method
4. Can be done comparative study in private and government hospital
5. Similar studies can be done on another age group.

FUTURE OVERVIEW

Achievable translatory component

The findings of this study can serve as the baseline information on the early onset of the sleep of hospitalized children in the selected areas of the study.

The findings are contributory to During pediatric hospitalization, sleep may be disrupted at a time when its advantages are most required. Frequent awakenings and short sleep duration have been shown to adversely impair a child's immunological response, pain perception, glucose management, and neuro endocrine function. Sleep deprivation causes diminished cognitive function, inattentive behavior, low attentiveness, and poor academic achievement in otherwise healthy youngsters.

Declaration of new knowledge generated

The purpose of this research was to get a effectiveness of a warm foot bath in promoting early sleep among hospitalised children. The BEARS (Children's scale for assessment of early onset of sleep). Sleep problems classified as BEARS are as follows: B=Breakdowns in sleep quality, E=Excessive Daytime Sleepiness, A=Night Awakenings, R=Regularity and Duration of Sleep, S=Snoring.

The tools generated from the present study may be applied for Copy write and can be utilized.

.The findings of the present study could be considered as a baseline and multi-area studies can be planned and executed.

The tools used for data collection can be used by nurses, student nurses of Child health nursing and community health department, and other health workers

3. Creating awareness among staff nurses and parents related to non-pharmacological intervention to improve the early sleep onset.

4. Warm foot bath helps to promote health of children.

It can reduce hospital stay of a child

Warm foot bath procedure can be used as a well defined guildline for the practices in hospital.

Summary

1. Lack of awareness regarding non-pharmacological intervention to improve the level of sleep among the population.
2. High incidence of sleep disturbance in hospitalized patient especially among the children.
3. There are no research studies that evaluated effect of warm foot bath on the early onset of sleep among children.

REFERENCES

1. Sleep [Internet]. The Nutrition Source. 2012 [cited 2022 May 20]. Available from: https://www.hsph.harvard.edu/nutritionsource/sleep/
2. Natural Patterns of Sleep | Healthy Sleep [Internet]. Healthysleep.med.harvard.edu. [cited 20 May 2022]. Available from: http://healthysleep.med.harvard.edu/healthy/science/what/sleep-patterns-rem-nrem
3. The Science of Sleep: Understanding What Happens When You Sleep [Internet]. Hopkinsmedicine.org. [cited 20 May 2022]. Available from: https://www.hopkinsmedicine.org/health/wellness-and-prevention/the-science-of-sleep-understanding-what-happens-when-you-sleep
4. Jung CM, Melanson EL, Frydendall EJ, Perreault L, Eckel RH, Wright KP. Energy expenditure during sleep, sleep deprivation and sleep following sleep deprivation in adult humans. The Journal of physiology. 2011 Jan 1;589(1):235-44.
5. Pagel JF. Nightmares and disorders of dreaming. American Family Physician. 2000 Apr 1;61(7):2037.
6. Kim TW, Jeong JH, Hong SC. The impact of sleep and circadian disturbance on hormones and metabolism. International journal of endocrinology. 2015 Oct;2015.
7. Hardin KA. Sleep in the ICU: potential mechanisms and clinical implications. Chest. 2009 Jul 1;136(1):284-94.
8. Hinds PS, Hockenberry M, Rai SN, Zhang L. Nocturnal awakenings, sleep environment interruptions, and fatigue in hospitalized children with cancer. InOncology nursing forum 2007 Mar 1; 34(2):393. Oncology Nursing Society.
9. Raghavan S. Here's why a foot bath will help you sleep like a baby [Internet]. The HealthSite. 2018 [cited 20 May 2022]. Available from: https://www.thehealthsite.com/diseases-conditions/insomnia/heres-why-a-foot-bath-will-help-you-sleep-like-a-baby-k0118-548476/
10. Fidler AL, Voorhees S, Zhou ES, Stacciarini JM, Fedele DA. A systematic review and proposed conceptual model of sleep disturbances during pediatric hospitalizations. Sleep. 2022 Feb 18.

11. Hybschmann J, Topperzer MK, Gjærde LK, Born P, Mathiasen R, Sehested AM, Jennum PJ, Sørensen JL. Sleep in hospitalized children and adolescents: A scoping review. Sleep medicine reviews. 2021 Oct 1;59:101496.
12. Farías-Fernández M, Rendón-Macías ME, Iglesias-Leboreiro J, Bernárdez-Zapata I, Gordillo-Rodríguez L. Effects of hospitalization on children's sleep pattern irrespective of sleep problems history. Boletínmédico del Hospital Infantil de México. 2021 Aug;78(4):279-86.
13. Crous EC, North N. Sleep promotion for hospitalised children: Developing an evidence-based guideline for nurses. curationis. 2021;44(1):1-0.
14. Sheikh IN, Roth M, Stavinoha PL. Prevalence of Sleep Disturbances in Pediatric Cancer Patients and Their Diagnosis and Management. Children. 2021 Dec;8(12):1100.
15. Sfeir E, Haddad C, Akel M, Hallit S, Obeid S. Sleep disorders in a sample of Lebanese children: the role of parental mental health and child nutrition and activity. BMC pediatrics. 2021 Dec;21(1):1-9.
16. Stremler R, Micsinszki S, Adams S, Parshuram C, Pullenayegum E, Weiss SK. Objective sleep characteristics and factors associated with sleep duration and waking during pediatric hospitalization. JAMA Network Open. 2021 Apr 1;4(4): e213924-.
17. Mainieri G, Montini A, Nicotera A, Di Rosa G, Provini F, Loddo G. The Genetics of Sleep Disorders in Children: A Narrative Review. Brain Sciences. 2021 Oct;11(10):1259.
18. Vecchi CR. Causes and effects of lack of sleep in hospitalized children. Arch Argent Pediatr. 2020 Apr 1;118(2):e143-7.
19. Herttrich T, Daxer J, Hiemisch A, Kluge J, Merkenschlager A, Kratzsch J, Scheuermann K, Jenni OG, Körner A, Kiess W, Quante M. Association of sleep characteristics with adiposity markers in children. Journal of Pediatric Endocrinology and Metabolism. 2020 Jul 1;33(7):845-52.
20. Erondu AI, Orlov NM, Peirce LB, Anderson SL, Chamberlain M, Hopkins K, Lyttle C, Gozal D, Arora VM. Characterizing pediatric inpatient sleep duration and disruptions. Sleep medicine. 2019 May 1;57:87-91.
21. Graef DM, Crabtree VM, Srivastava DK, Li C, Pritchard M, Hinds PS, Mandrell B. Sleep and mood during hospitalization for high- dose

chemotherapy and hematopoietic rescue in pediatric medulloblastoma. Psycho- Oncology. 2018 Jul;27(7):1847-53.

22. Lee S, Narendran G, Tomfohr- Madsen L, Schulte F. A systematic review of sleep in hospitalized pediatric cancer patients. Psycho- oncology. 2017 Aug;26(8):1059-69.
23. Stickland A, Clayton E, Sankey R, Hill CM. A qualitative study of sleep quality in children and their resident parents when in hospital. Archives of disease in childhood. 2016 Jun 1;101(6):546-51.
24. Bisogni S, Chiarini I, Giusti F, Ciofi D, Poggi GM, Festini F. Impact of hospitalization on the sleep patterns of newborns, infants and toddlers admitted to a pediatric ward: a cross-sectional study. Minerva pediatrica. 2014 Oct 9;67(3):209-17.
25. Snodgrass K, Harvey A, Scheinberg A, Knight S. Sleep disturbances in pediatric chronic fatigue syndrome: a review of current research. Journal of Clinical Sleep Medicine. 2015 Jul 15;11(7):757-64.
26. Herbert AR, De Lima J, Fitzgerald DA, Seton C, Waters KA, Collins JJ. Exploratory study of sleeping patterns in children admitted to hospital. Journal of paediatrics and child health. 2014 Aug;50(8):632-8.
27. Meltzer LJ, Avis KT, Biggs S, Reynolds AC, Crabtree VM, Bevans KB. The Children's Report of Sleep Patterns (CRSP): a self-report measure of sleep for school-aged children. Journal of Clinical Sleep Medicine. 2013 Mar 15;9(3):235-45.
28. Linder LA, Christian BJ. Nighttime sleep disruptions, the hospital care environment, and symptoms in elementary school-age children with cancer. InOncology nursing forum 2012 Nov (Vol. 39, No. 6, p. 553). NIH Public Access.
29. Hall WA, Scher A, Zaidman- Zait A, Espezel H, Warnock F. A community- based study of sleep and behaviour problems in 12- to 36- month- old children. Child: care, health and development. 2012 May;38(3):379-89.
30. Byars KC, Yolton K, Rausch J, Lanphear B, Beebe DW. Prevalence, patterns, and persistence of sleep problems in the first 3 years of life. Pediatrics. 2012 Feb 1;129(2):e276-84.

31. Spruyt K, Gozal D. Sleep disturbances in children with attention-deficit/hyperactivity disorder. Expert review of neurotherapeutics. 2011 Apr 1;11(4):565-77.
32. Jenni OG, LeBourgeois MK. Understanding sleep–wake behavior and sleep disorders in children: the value of a model. Current opinion in psychiatry. 2006 May;19(3):282.
33. Davis KF, Parker KP, Montgomery GL. Sleep in infants and young children: part two: common sleep problems. Journal of Pediatric Health Care. 2004 May 1;18(3):130-7.
34. Stein MA, Mendelsohn J, Obermeyer WH, Amromin J, Benca R. Sleep and behavior problems in school-aged children. Pediatrics. 2001 Apr 1;107(4):e60-.
35. Thiedke CC. Sleep disorders and sleep problems in childhood. American Family Physician. 2001 Jan 15;63(2):277.
36. Owens JA, Spirito A, McGuinn M, Nobile C. Sleep habits and sleep disturbance in elementary school-aged children. Journal of Developmental and Behavioral Pediatrics. 2000 Feb 1;21(1):27-36.
37. Ho KY, Lam KK, Xia W, Chung JO, Cheung AT, Ho LL, Chiu SY, Chan GC, Li WH. Psychometric properties of the Chinese version of the Pittsburgh Sleep Quality Index (PSQI) among Hong Kong Chinese childhood cancer survivors. Health and Quality of Life Outcomes. 2021 Dec;19(1):1-1.
38. Larche CL, Plante I, Roy M, Ingelmo PM, Ferland CE. The Pittsburgh Sleep Quality Index: Reliability, factor structure, and related clinical factors among children, adolescents, and young adults with chronic pain. Sleep disorders. 2021 Apr 26;2021.
39. Panzarella V, Giuliana G, Spinuzza P, La Mantia G, Maniscalco L, Pizzo G, Matranga D. Paediatric Sleep Questionnaire for Obstructive Sleep Apnoea Syndrome Screening: Is Sleep Quality Worthy of Note?. Applied Sciences. 2021 Jan;11(4):1440.
40. Romeo DM, Cordaro G, Macchione E, Venezia I, Brogna C, Mercuri E, Bruni O. Application of the Sleep Disturbance Scale for Children (SDSC) in infants and toddlers (6–36 months). Sleep medicine. 2021 May 1;81:62-8.

41. Moo-Estrella JA, Valencia-Flores M, Arankowsky-Sandoval GM. Development and validation of the Sleep Disturbances Scale for School-age Children. Acta pediátrica de México. 2018 Apr;39(2):121-33.
42. Erwin AM, Bashore L. Subjective sleep measures in children: self-report. Frontiers in pediatrics. 2017 Feb 13;5:22.
43. Üçer O, Gümüş B. Quantifying subjective assessment of sleep quality, quality of life and depressed mood in children with enuresis. World journal of urology. 2014 Feb;32(1):239-43.
44. Simola P, Laitalainen E, Liukkonen K, Virkkula P, Kirjavainen T, Pitkäranta A, Aronen ET. Sleep disturbances in a community sample from preschool to school age. Child: care, health and development. 2012 Jul;38(4):572-80.
45. Sohn SI, Kim DH, Lee MY, Cho YW. The reliability and validity of the Korean version of the Pittsburgh Sleep Quality Index. Sleep and Breathing. 2012 Sep;16(3):803-12.
46. Waumans RC, Terwee CB, Van den Berg G, Knol DL, Van Litsenburg RR, Gemke RJ. Sleep and sleep disturbance in children: Reliability and validity of the Dutch version of the Child Sleep Habits Questionnaire. Sleep. 2010 Jun 1;33(6):841-5.
47. Spruyt K, Gozal D. Pediatric sleep questionnaires as diagnostic or epidemiological tools: a review of currently available instruments. Sleep medicine reviews. 2011 Feb 1;15(1):19-32.
48. Ertan P, Yilmaz O, Caglayan M, Sogut A, Aslan S, Yuksel H. Relationship of sleep quality and quality of life in children with monosymptomatic enuresis. Child: care, health and development. 2009 Jul;35(4):469-74.
49. Ferreira VR, Carvalho LB, Ruotolo F, de Morais JF, Prado LB, Prado GF. Sleep disturbance scale for children: translation, cultural adaptation, and validation. Sleep medicine. 2009 Apr 1;10(4):457-63.
50. Goodlin-Jones BL, Sitnick SL, Tang K, Liu J, Anders TF. The Children's Sleep Habits Questionnaire in toddlers and preschool children. Journal of Developmental & Behavioral Pediatrics. 2008 Apr 1;29(2):82-8.
51. Narendhran R, Bharti B, Malhi P. Children Sleep Habits Question-naire (CSHQ): psychometric validation in Indian school children. Indian J Sleep Med. 2008;3.

52. Melendres CS, Lutz JM, Rubin ED, Marcus CL. Daytime sleepiness and hyperactivity in children with suspected sleep-disordered breathing. Pediatrics. 2004 Sep 1;114(3):768-75.
53. Drake C, Nickel C, Burduvali E, Roth T, Jefferson C, Badia P. The pediatric daytime sleepiness scale (PDSS): sleep habits and school outcomes in middle-school children. Sleep. 2003 Jun 1;26(4):455-8.
54. Backhaus J, Junghanns K, Broocks A, Riemann D, Hohagen F. Test–retest reliability and validity of the Pittsburgh Sleep Quality Index in primary insomnia. Journal of psychosomatic research. 2002 Sep 1;53(3):737-40.
55. Chervin RD, Hedger K, Dillon JE, Pituch KJ. Pediatric sleep questionnaire (PSQ): validity and reliability of scales for sleep-disordered breathing, snoring, sleepiness, and behavioral problems. Sleep medicine. 2000 Feb 1;1(1):21-32.
56. Bruni O, Ottaviano S, Guidetti V, Romoli M, Innocenzi M, Cortesi F, Giannotti F. The Sleep Disturbance Scale for Children (SDSC) Construct ion and validation of an instrument to evaluate sleep disturbances in childhood and adolescence. Journal of sleep research. 1996 Dec;5(4):251-61.
57. Chen X, ling Ke Z, Chen Y, Lin X. The prevalence of sleep problems among children in mainland China: a meta-analysis and systemic-analysis. Sleep Medicine. 2021 Jul 1;83:248-55.
58. Haghayegh S, Khoshnevis S, Smolensky MH, Diller KR, Castriotta RJ. Before-bedtime passive body heating by warm shower or bath to improve sleep: A systematic review and meta-analysis. Sleep medicine reviews. 2019 Aug 1;46:124-35.
59. Cayuelas LM, March-Villalba JA, Guadalajara VV, Durbá AS, Baenas MC, Rodrigo AP, Hinarejos CD, Tormo FB. Evaluation of sleep hygiene and prevalence of sleep disorders in patients with monosymptomatic enuresis. Usefulness of the BEARS sleep screening tool. ActasUrológicasEspañolas (English Edition). 2020 Sep 1;44(7):477-82.
60. Ramirez-Velez R, Huertas-Zamora L, Correa-Bautista JE, Cárdenas-Calderón EG. Reliability and validity of the BEARS sleep disorder questionnaire in children and adolescent students from Bogotá, DC, Colombia: FUPRECOL study. 2018.

61. Peter ID, Adamu H, Asani MO, Aliyu I, Sabo UA, Umar UI. Sleep pattern and sleep hygiene practices among Nigerian schooling adolescents. Indian journal of psychological medicine. 2017 Jul;39(4):407-12.
62. Bagalkot PS, Mayur SS. Sleep Problems among Rural Preschool Aged Children.International Journal of Health Sciences & Research. 2017;7(8)
63. Bastida- Pozuelo MF, Sanchez- Ortuno MM. Preliminary analysis of the concurrent validity of the Spanish translation of the BEARS sleep screening tool for children. Journal of Psychiatric and Mental Health Nursing. 2016 Oct;23(8):513-20.
64. Javadi, M., Javadi, A., Kalantari, N., Jaliloghadr, S., & Mohamad, H. (2014). Sleep Problems among Pre-School Children in Qazvin, Iran. *The Malaysian journal of medical sciences : MJMS*, *21*(6), 52–56.
65. Bharti B, Mehta A, Malhi P. Sleep problems in children: A guide for primary care physicians. The Indian Journal of Pediatrics. 2013 Jun;80(6):492-8.
66. Amintehran E, Ghalehbaghi B, Asghari A, Jalilolghadr S, Ahmadvand A, Foroughi F. High prevalence of sleep problems in school-and preschool-aged children in Tehran: a population based study. Iranian journal of pediatrics. 2013 Feb;23(1):45.
67. Peter ID, Adamu H, Asani MO, Aliyu I, Sabo UA, Umar UI. Sleep pattern and sleep hygiene practices among Nigerian schooling adolescents. Indian journal of psychological medicine. 2017 Jul;39(4):407-12.
68. Shahid A, Wilkinson K, Marcu S, Shapiro CM. BEARS sleep screening tool. InSTOP, THAT and One Hundred Other Sleep Scales 2011 (pp. 59-61). Springer, New York, NY.
69. Ravikiran SR, Jagadeesh Kumar PM, Latha KS. Sleep problems in preschool and school aged rural Indian children. Indian pediatrics. 2011 Mar;48(3):221-3.
70. Mohammadi M, Ebrahim Amintehran MF, Ghaleh-bandi MR, Shoaee S, Ghalehbaghi B. Reliability and validity of Persian version of "BEARS" pediatric sleep questionnaire. Indian Journal of Sleep Medicine (IJSM). 2008;3(1).

71. Owens JA, Dalzell V. Use of the 'BEARS'sleep screening tool in a pediatric residents' continuity clinic: a pilot study. Sleep medicine. 2005 Jan 1;6(1):63-9.10
72. Semiz M, Uslu A, Korkmaz S, Demir S, Parlak I, Sencan M, Aydin B, Uncu T. Assessment of subjective sleep quality in iron deficiency anaemia. African health sciences. 2015;15(2):621-7.
73. Halstead EJ, Joyce A, Sullivan E, Tywyn C, Davies K, Jones A, Dimitriou D. Sleep disturbances and patterns in children with neurodevelopmental conditions. Frontiers in pediatrics. 2021 Mar 2; 9:91.
74. Narasimhan U, Anitha FS, Anbu C. The spectrum of sleep disorders among children: a cross-sectional study at a South Indian tertiary care hospital. Cureus. 2020 Apr 4;12(4).
75. Merz EL, Tomfohr-Madsen L. Sleep disruption in pediatric cancer survivors: Conceptual framework and opportunities for clinical assessment and behavioral treatment. American Journal of Lifestyle Medicine. 2018 Jul;12(4):311-23.
76. Rabner J, Kaczynski KJ, Simons LE, LeBel A. Pediatric headache and sleep disturbance: a comparison of diagnostic groups. Headache: The Journal of Head and Face Pain. 2018 Feb;58(2):217-28.
77. Hale L, Guan S. Screen time and sleep among school-aged children and adolescents: a systematic literature review. Sleep medicine reviews. 2015 Jun 1;21:50-8.
78. Lewandowski AS, Ward TM, Palermo TM. Sleep problems in children and adolescents with common medical conditions. Pediatric Clinics. 2011 Jun 1;58(3):699-713.
79. Heyer GL, Rose SC, Merison K, Perkins SQ, Lee JE. Specific headache factors predict sleep disturbances among youth with migraine. Pediatric Neurology. 2014 Oct 1;51(4):489-93.
80. Orsey AD, Wakefield DB, Cloutier MM. Physical activity (PA) and sleep among children and adolescents with cancer. Pediatric blood & cancer. 2013 Nov;60(11):1908-13.
81. Dosi C, Riccioni A, Della Corte M, Novelli L, Ferri R, Bruni O. Comorbidities of sleep disorders in childhood and adolescence: focus on migraine. Nature and Science of Sleep. 2013; 5:77.

82. Alfano CA, Kim KL. Objective sleep patterns and severity of symptoms in pediatric obsessive compulsive disorder: a pilot investigation. Journal of anxiety disorders. 2011 Aug 1;25(6):835-9.
83. Bell J Zimmerman FJ. Shortened nighttime sleep duration in early life and subsequent childhood obesity. Archives of pediatrics& adolescent medicine. 2010 Sep 1;164(9):840-5.
84. Chokroverty S. Overview of sleep & sleep disorders. Indian J Med Res. 2010 Feb 1;131(2):126-40.
85. Hysing M, Sivertsen B, Stormark KM, Elgen I, Lundervold AJ. Sleep in children with chronic illness, and the relation to emotional and behavioral problems—a population-based study. Journal of Pediatric Psychology. 2009 Jul 1;34(6):665-70.
86. Sivertsen B, Hysing M, Elgen I, Stormark KM, Lundervold AJ. Chronicity of sleep problems in children with chronic illness: a longitudinal population-based study. Child and adolescent psychiatry and mental health. 2009 Dec;3(1):1-7.
87. Stores G. Aspects of sleep disorders in children and adolescents. *Dialogues ClinNeurosci*. 2009;11(1):81-90.
88. Long AC, Krishnamurthy V, Palermo TM. Sleep disturbances in school-age children with chronic pain. Journal of pediatric psychology. 2008 Apr 1;33(3):258-68.
89. Hart CN, Jelalian E. Shortened sleep duration is associated with pediatric overweight. Behavioral sleep medicine. 2008 Oct 21;6(4):251-67.
90. Isik U, Ersu RH, Ay P, Save D, Arman AR, Karakoc F, Dagli E. Prevalence of headache and its association with sleep disorders in children. Pediatric neurology. 2007 Mar 1;36(3):146-51.
91. Fricke-Oerkermann L, Plück J, Schredl M, Heinz K, Mitschke A, Wiater A, Lehmkuhl G. Prevalence and course of sleep problems in childhood. Sleep. 2007 Oct 1;30(10):1371-7.
92. Smaldone A, Honig JC, Byrne MW. Sleepless in America: inadequate sleep and relationships to health and well-being of our nation's children. Pediatrics. 2007 Feb 1;119(Supplement_1): S29-37.

93. Russo PM, Bruni O, Lucidi F, Ferri R, Violani C. Sleep habits and circadian preference in Italian children and adolescents. Journal of sleep research. 2007 Jun;16(2):163-9.

94. Luc ME, Gupta A, Birnberg JM, Reddick D, Kohrman MH. Characterization of symptoms of sleep disorders in children with headache. Pediatric neurology. 2006 Jan 1;34(1):7-12.

95. Heng K, Wirrell E. Sleep disturbance in children with migraine. Journal of Child Neurology. 2006 Sep;21(9):761-6.

96. Carotenuto M, Guidetti V, Ruju F, Galli F, Tagliente FR, Pascotto A. Headache disorders as risk factors for sleep disturbances in school aged children. The Journal of Headache and Pain. 2005 Sep;6(4):268-70.

97. Miller VA, Palermo TM, Powers SW, Scher MS, Hershey A. Migraine headaches and sleep disturbances in children. Headache: The Journal of Head and Face Pain. 2003 Apr;43(4):362-8.

98. Mohamad SS, Ahmed SM, Tawfic AH, Nagaty A. Effect of Warm Water Foot Bath Therapy on Body Temperature among Children with Fever. SYLWAN. 2021 Feb;165(2)

99. El-Naggar NS, Mohamed HR. Effectiveness of Warm Water Footbath on Temperature and Fatigue among Children with Fever. Evidence-Based Nursing Research. 2020;2(4):11-

100. .Pereira AC, Sebastian S. Effectiveness of hot water foot bath therapy inreduction of temperature among children (6-12 years)with fever in selected hospitals at Mangaluru. Int J Appl Res. 2018; 4:86-92.

101. Mandal I, Datta S, Ahmed N, De P. Effectiveness of Warm Water Foot-Bath Therapy on Physiological Parameters of Children with Fever at a Selected Hospital, Kolkata, West Bengal. Journal of Nursing Science & Practice. 2014;4(2):43-57.

CPSIA information can be obtained
at www.ICGtesting.com
Printed in the USA
LVHW022049140423
744403LV00010B/499

9 788993 218312